THE ART OF RUNNING

WITH THE ALEXANDER TECHNIQUE

MALCOLM BALK &
ANDREW SHIELDS

ASHGROVE PUBLISHING
LONDON & BATH

IN MEMORY OF
HUGO REIMER BALK

CONTENTS

ACKNOWLEDGEMENTS

I would like to thank all my fellow Alexander Technique teachers, with particular gratitude to Robin Simmons, director of the Hampstead Alexander Centre, for his vision, energy and support. Also to Shoshana Kaminitz and the late Patrick Macdonald for creating the chance for me to become a teacher of the Technique.

A big kiss to everyone who wrote a testimony or allowed themselves to be a case study for this book. To my friend Doreen for her feedback at our weekly breakfast meetings: the next one's on me. And to Dave, Tina and Dougal for providing great company and a base on the Grove.

Un gros merci à Bernard Godbout pour tout son inspiration comme entraineur. I'd also like to thank Patrick Denis for helping with the computer and Patrick McDonaugh for his feedback on the manuscript.

Finally, a special thank you to my wife Pamela for her love and support.

Malcolm Balk

Thanks to Paola Corteen at the Westminster Alexander Centre for her patience in trying to coax my body into a state of 'balanced rest'; and to her colleague John Hunter, for many useful observations on the manuscript. The staff, volunteers and members at Central YMCA deserve gratitude not only for keeping me in shape, but for help with photographic ideas during the very early stages of the book – Uta Saatz, in particular. A special thanks to Steven Shaw for his constant encouragement; to Richard Francis and his staff at Action Plus for their great photos; and to Tim Everson of Kingston Museum and Heritage Service for assistance with the Muybridge pictures.

As the London link in this trans-Atlantic project, my dealings with Brad Thompson of Ashgrove Publishing were unfailingly enthusiastic. And it would all have been a lot harder had my wife Elaine, and children Helen, Isabel and Matthew, not been so understanding whenever daddy said he needed to 'disappear' into his study for an hour or two...

Andrew Shields

INTRODUCTION

This book gives me a chance to talk about two favourite subjects: running and the Alexander Technique. It is safe to say that the continued enjoyment I gain from the sport is due in no small measure to the influence of a remarkable man, Frederick Matthias Alexander (1869–1955), and the fact that in 1979 I was introduced to the Alexander Technique by my cello teacher, bless her heart.

Since becoming an Alexander Technique teacher, I have been able to correct the poor form of those who ran much as I once did – by putting one foot in front of the other as fast as possible and, if running on a track, turning left occasionally. When I took up running in the mid-1970s, my interest was primarily competitive. Although I enjoyed training, my main aim was to reduce the time it took to complete a 10k race or a marathon. Despite aches, pains and a general lack of raw talent, I grew to love the sport and kept looking for ways to get better. But as I describe elsewhere in this book, my somewhat narrow definition of improvement brought less and less satisfaction. In fact, my progress as a runner almost came to a complete halt when, plagued by injury and a disappointing result in the Ottawa Marathon, I thought seriously about quitting and finding something else to do.

My passion for the sport was rekindled by a chance encounter with a great coach, who focused on form first and performance second. This meeting and subsequent friendship fuelled a deeper desire to learn more about improving human performance.

The great athlete Filbert Bayi once said: 'From running I derive not just physical but aesthetic pleasure'. It is worth considering what he meant, and also what the title of this book means: *The Art of Running*. Our experience of art is usually limited to the end product: we attend the concert, admire the painting, read the book – or, just as validly, leap from our seats at the end of a thrilling track final. We all want to share the moment, although our involvement is inevitably restricted to that of an onlooker.

How, then, can we feel more involved with the creative process? We may not be able to conduct an orchestra, pen a best-seller or win an Olympic gold medal, but we can do something else which is common to all top musicians, writers, dancers, artists and athletes: that is, to practise. After all, we do speak of practising as an art.

Wilson Kipketer won the 1999 World Championships 800m final in 1 min 42 secs, but it took him 15, maybe even 20, years of practice to do so: a period spent partly in the company of his fellow runners, but mostly by himself. What can we bring to our practice that will give it a different quality compared to what my Alexander teacher, Patrick Macdonald, referred to as 'mindless repetition like the heathens'?

When running becomes a means to an end – be it fitness, fame or fat reduction – it loses the features which elevate it from just another mundane activity. It's a bit like the difference between painting your bathroom and painting a portrait of your true love: both use paint and a brush, but the first is an exercise in utilitarianism, the second an act of creation.

However, running can very easily become like painting your bathroom. When we cut our minds off from what we are doing and simply repeat a learned gesture mechanically over and over, without interest or curiosity, without thought, without intention and without humanity, we reduce both the experience and ourselves in the process. We are no longer in the flow zone, we are in ozone. The focus shifts from a childlike immersion in the moment, to simply 'getting it done'.

While this is not intended as a conventional 'how to' book, there are chapters which show how some of the procedures used in Alexander Technique can facilitate awareness and good form in the runner. The aim is to explore the discoveries made by Alexander and how they relate to the art of running, and to set this kind of work within the wider context of fitness, sport and exercise going into the 21st century. The chapter on competition discusses some of the dangers as well as the joys associated with this approach to running. Note also that, unless stated otherwise, 'I' in the text refers to Malcolm Balk.

The art of running is to be found in the process, in the act itself. Where else can it be found? The beauty of this art is that it can (indeed, it has to) be recreated every time you run, in every step you take, as Sting put it. It doesn't matter what you did yesterday, or even what you did two minutes ago – it's the next step that counts.

I hope this book will help you find your place on the path, and that our routes will one day cross.

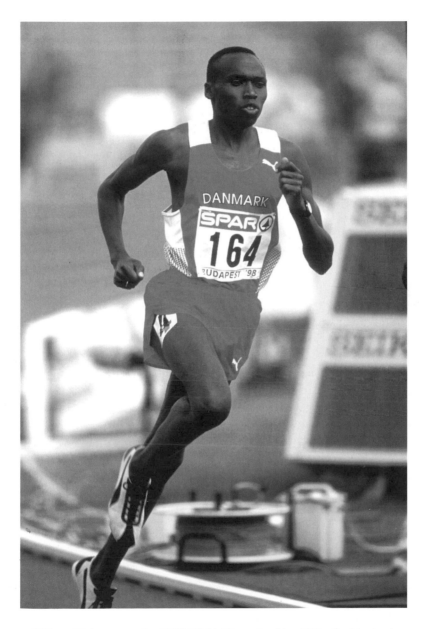

Wilson Kipketer won the 1999 World Championships 800m final in 1 min 42 secs, but it may have taken 15, even 20, years of practice to enable him to do so.

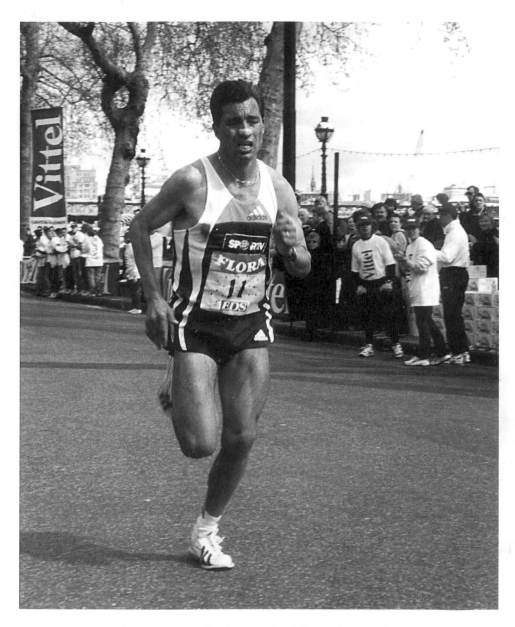

Antonio Pinto maintains control and focus as he nears the
finishing line of the 2000 Flora London Marathon.

1. MASTERING THE ART

Like any art, mastering the tools of the trade is an important step towards enjoying the process. Learning to run takes time, energy and consistency: you have to do it regularly to become good at it. And until you've achieved a certain level of competence, it is unlikely that you will enjoy it very much, or for very long. When I tell runners that there is something new to be learned every time they put on their shoes, they look at me with scepticism and sometimes disbelief. But the truth is that, even though I've been running for more than 25 years, I still feel like I learn something every day. It's not just a cliché, it's what feeds the process. Being curious about what we are doing is another key component of practising an art – without it, everything gets old, stale, lifeless. And there is always something to learn. If world record-holders can comment that they could have done better if they'd had a smoother start, or had been more relaxed or more focused, then the rest of us can certainly find something to discover, change or improve. As Alexander himself put it: 'Control must be in the process, not superimposed'.

Even when running is hard – as it often is when I'm tired or trying to achieve a particular target in training – I find that renewing my sense of wonder at being able to express who I am in this way changes the experience from a job to a joy. Being passionate about what you practise is one of the keys to making something an art.

I like to run. I feel good when I run (most of the time). I enjoy it even more now that I am getting better at recognising when I'm running for the wrong reasons, such as: because I'm supposed to, because it's Monday, because I have to maintain an image or prove something, because I have to fill in my diary. But also when I'm running for the right reasons: to enjoy the feeling of movement, to overcome inertia and begin to flow, to think, to do battle with my demons, to transcend the elements, to renew myself, to connect with the beauty and energy and greatness that running in all its forms represents. And most important of all, just for the hell of it!

In a book entitled *A Year of Living Consciously*, Gay Hendricks poses the question: 'What if you invested every action you take with lovingness and creativity?' The quotation he includes with that day's entry is from Picasso: 'Every child is an artist. The problem is how to remain an artist once he grows up.'

One of the trends I have noticed in running and fitness during the 1990s and into the new millennium is that it has become a job. It is serious business. For some people this attains religious proportions. Miss a workout? Go straight to hell, or purgatory at least! You see these types out there, poodling along at ten minutes per mile, hooked in to their Walkman, a fanatical look in their eyes, as if to say: 'Don't talk to me now, can't you see I'm *training*?' When any activity becomes routine, no matter what it is, boredom and blindness set in and we wish we were somewhere else doing something more exciting.

When I began working with musicians, I was amazed to discover how many professional musicians seemed to dislike music! Comments like: 'Oh, God, not Beethoven *again!*' were not unusual.

How did this happen? How could it have been prevented? And if it can happen to playing Beethoven, what chance do ironing, cooking and running have?

One of the early signs that an activity is becoming routine is a tendency to distance yourself from what you are doing. By 'distance' I don't mean a healthy detachment which allows you to see what is going on with greater clarity, less interference and more control. I'm talking about the semi-comatose, trance-like state we can easily slide into, especially when we are doing something we've done a thousand times before. Remember the first time you got behind the wheel of a car? I can still recall the excitement of putting the vehicle into gear and steering around a vacant parking lot. Is driving anything like that today?

Or the first time you made love? More predictable now, is it? Or the start of your first marathon? Wow, I've never heard so much yelling and cheering! Do you still experience any of that when you are out there running?

I used to react rather defensively when people would say: 'Oh, you run. Don't you find it a bit boring?' Well, the fact of the matter is that if sex and music can become a little ho-hum, then running certainly can, too.

Alexander offers us a way out of this malaise. He believed that when we become overly pre-occupied with results, we lose touch with the process, what he called the 'means whereby'. This self-limiting attitude is so widespread in our society that it could almost be called normal (although certainly not natural). Getting back in touch with the process puts us in the moment, each of which is a little different from the one before.

Assuming that we know how to run, for example, is one way of stopping what should be an ongoing process of learning and discovery. You say you've been running for ten years and, by golly, you ought to know what you're doing by now. Yet this kind of thinking leaves you bankrupt, as far as learning goes. I have yet to work with a runner who didn't have something that could be improved or changed, be it more speed, fewer injuries, better form and more fun!

Alexander wrote that 'The experience you want is in the getting of it. If you have something, give it up. Getting it, not having it, is what you want.' As a competitive athlete, I know how hard it is to hold on to good form. In fact, trying to hold on to it makes it worse. With the Alexander Technique, the process of letting go, only to find again anew, is something we live with each day.

Every run is different, and how I react to each run can be a matter of choice, or creation. As I run today, I notice that my right hamstring feels tight, that there is a chill in the air, and I sense it might snow. As I run up the mountain I am monitoring my leg, and also noting how it is affecting my overall form. It has caused me to tighten in my back and run a bit more heavily than I would wish. So I decide to stop and give my body some purposeful direction. I point myself upwards, encourage my knees and ankles to release, and start again. It is already better: the stride is smoother and I am breathing more freely. One hundred metres further on, I stop once more and repeat the process. As I pick up pace, I notice that my hamstring is starting to release, but still has the occasional twinge. I continue, but later, as I am doing some accelerations, I note that my hamstring has let go and is now part of my overall sense of falling upward and forward. I press on with the day's workout, taking care not to let its demands overwhelm my kinaesthetic ear and my decision to flow rather than force my way through each repetition.

That is an example of what I consider running as an act of creativity: staying present, responding intelligently to the situation, taking calculated risks, finding a different way to achieve your goal. I had completed a version of that workout many times over the years, but on that particular autumn day, it was an experience that demanded my creative intelligence to tackle it.

Was it boring? Hardly. Finding a way to run up a hill ten times without damaging myself was a major accomplishment. It was not simply a matter of will. Now I am into my 40s, pain wins just about every time. I can't 'muscle' my way through tough workouts any more. But I still enjoy the feeling of pushing myself hard, working up a good sweat, and teasing younger athletes when they start to whine about how gruelling it is to run up that damn hill ten times – as in,

'Well, you know, the first nine times are the toughest'. Maybe that's one of the blessings of getting older. If you want to keep doing some of the things you love, you simply have to get more creative.

My story – Malcolm Balk

In 1974, I made two decisions which changed my life. First, I quit playing ice hockey. Second, I decided to take up two new and seemingly unrelated activities: playing the cello and running.

I have always loved sport, and particularly ice hockey from the first time I saw it being played on an outdoor rink when I was aged seven. For the next 13 years it was an all-consuming passion. This pursuit, which I dreamed would end up with me playing for the Montreal Canadians, was briefly interrupted in High School when my mother made me take cello lessons. But after a year I gave this up to focus on ice hockey, which by then I was playing at a reasonably serious level. However, as I grew less and less fond of getting beaten up and the fantasy of playing in the big leagues began to fade, a serious knee injury encouraged me to quit. And at that point, I knew immediately that I really wanted to play the cello again.

There's an old Yiddish joke that goes something like: 'Do you know how to play the violin?' Answer: 'Don't know, never tried'. Well, I found myself a cello teacher and tried like hell to learn how to play, but the harder I tried the worse it got. At least with ice hockey, if you got a little tense you could go out on the rink and hit somebody. With the cello, that kind of release just wasn't acceptable. And so, I found myself in a bind where I knew there was a better cellist in me striving to get out, but the kind of effort and tension I was making in the process seemed to block any progress. For the sake of my sanity and my neighbours' ears, I needed to find a solution. But what?

Parallel to my trials and tribulations with the cello was a growing interest and increased participation in running. As a competitive athlete, I had always run – as part of playing baseball and Canadian football, and once a year in the High School track and field meeting. In 1975, the running boom was in full swing – and when my girlfriend declared her intention to run a marathon, I was stricken in more ways than one!

Over the next five years I completed five marathons, and managed to suffer a wide range of injuries common to many fellow distance runners: achilles tendonitis, runner's knee, shin splints, calf, quad and hamstring pulls, and more. Although I managed to improve my times, there was a growing sense of concern with a pattern that was becoming more apparent. As I put more and more effort and mileage into running, I seemed to get less back. Many runners are familiar with the thinking that underlies this problem: if I run a marathon in 2 hr 50 mins on 50 miles a week, then when I push my mileage to 70 miles a week I'll run the same distance in 2 hr 40 mins. If only it was that simple. I had discovered the Law of Diminishing Returns, and more was turning into less. So there I was, stuck again.

Two things happened which pointed the way forward. First, I met Bernard Godbout, a running coach who talked about learning how to run. Not just go easy on Mondays, harder on Tuesdays and harder still at the weekend, but to think about form: in other words, what your knees were doing, how to use your arms when you wanted to accelerate, and so on. After meeting Bernard I decided to go back to basics, starting with how to run the 100 metres.

Around this time, my cello teacher returned from a trip to London very excited about something called Alexander Technique. Her enthusiasm convinced several of her students, me included, to begin taking lessons. These, combined with reading Dr Wilfred Barlow's book *The Alexander Principle*, led me to the following conclusion: in order to improve, be it at the cello or on the track, I had to rid myself of habits which were constantly interfering with my ability to play like Rostropovich or run like Sebastian Coe.

In 1981, I moved to London to begin training to become an Alexander Technique teacher. For three hours every morning we would meet at the school near Victoria, run by Patrick Macdonald. It was an exciting period, when I and my fellow trainees struggled to make sense of Alexander's teachings and to learn to apply them to our lives. I took my cello with me, and also kept up my running, now focusing on the 800 metres. Some teachers insist that their pupils cease vigorous activity until they have sufficiently integrated the principles of the Technique, for fear that the muscular effort involved will be counter-productive to their training. I discussed this with Macdonald, who gave me permission to keep running on the proviso that I did not get myself into a state. This inspired me to become aware of how I was running.

And it was here that I felt the first effects of Alexander work. Although my weekly load included several tough interval training sessions, the sort of track work familiar to every middle-distance runner, there was a big difference. I was no longer plagued with injuries. Furthermore, my times kept getting

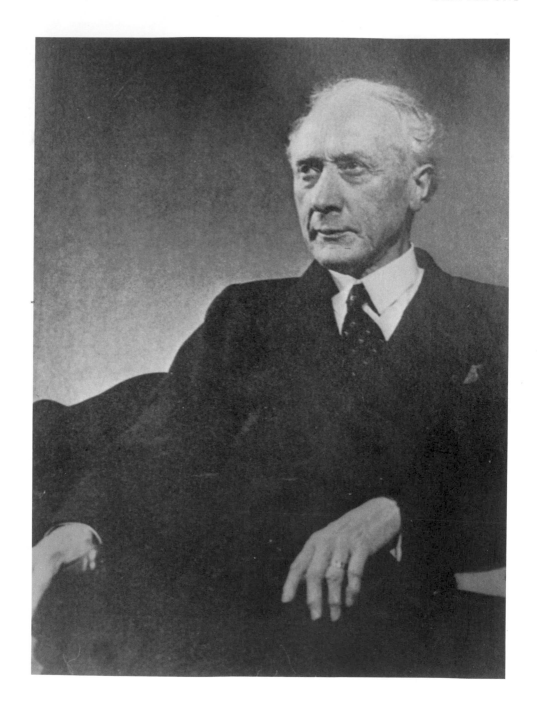

faster right into my late 30s and now, in my early 40s, I maintain a level close to my personal bests. And still, no injuries. Coincidentally, with the help of a fellow teacher who was also a cellist, music became much less of a trial and more of a pleasure.

Several themes emerged from this process: to improve, one needs to know what to do, how to do it and what not to do. My studies began to equip me with a 'kinaesthetic conscience'. In other words, I became much more aware of how I did everything, from the way I sat, to how I tied my shoes, to how I reached for my pint of beer. Up to this point, I, like many runners, was completely unaware of the warning signals which occurred when I trained. These ranged from small aches and pains, to staleness and cold symptoms. My typical response, through sheer force of will or perhaps what Alexander called 'stupidity in living', was simply to train through them. However, my studies taught me that I could no longer overlook these signs, or dismiss them as inconsequential.

Alexander said that happiness was being able to do something you loved to do, well. For me, this created a passion to learn how to run well – a passion which still burns today. In the Alexander Technique, we emphasise learning how to achieve more with less, how to 'get out of the way and let it happen'. Now this expression may seem a little esoteric, but to me it indicated a direction, a way of running that included and went beyond just 'doing it'.

Fast forward to 1988. Now a qualified teacher, I attended the International Alexander Technique Conference in Brighton. There, several participants, hearing that I was a runner, asked me to work with them. In doing so, it soon became obvious that the Technique could be extremely useful in helping runners to become more aware of and reduce their bad habits, as well as improve their form. And, of course, have a lot of fun in the process.

Three years later I had developed a more organised workshop applying Alexander's principles and procedures to running. This basic format has since been refined, but its essence remains the same: runners of all standards, from beginners to élites, can improve their form and, with luck, their performances. In practical terms, too, this approach to running has had a very important benefit. Over 16 years of regular training and competition for the 800 metres, I did not suffer a single serious injury.

Opposite: *Frederick Matthias Alexander (1869-1955).*

MY STORY – ANDREW SHIELDS

My serious athletics career ended painfully at the age of 19 – with a fractured lumbar vertebra after a triple jump went from hop to step to collapse. Despite reaching three English Schools finals and gaining a national junior ranking, I was not too disappointed; cricket was my other main summer interest, and it was obvious that, once I had left home and lost access to parents willing to shuttle me uncomplainingly between venues, I would need to choose between the two activities. Injury treated, I continued competing at university – but in a more half-hearted fashion, with the thought that I could sustain similar damage always at the back of my mind. Thereafter, I 'retired' from track and field to concentrate on cricket, while taking up another biomechanically suspect sport, hockey.

I began to make my way in sports journalism, eventually becoming sports editor of *Time Out* in 1990. I expanded this role to include writing about fitness, health and personal development, which gave me the chance to try a wide range of complementary therapies and what were still considered 'alternative' practices: numerous massage techniques, reflexology, reiki, flotation, yoga, tai chi, Pilates and so on. It was interesting to relate these to sport and explore how athletes from every background could benefit — a link which few practitioners at the time had made. Only recently, for example, have tennis and cricket coaches discovered the relevance and usefulness of tai chi.

It was through sport that I came upon the Alexander Technique. I heard about Steven Shaw's work linking the Technique with swimming (see Chapter 3), and went for lessons. Although I could swim reasonable distances, my technique was poor. I envied those sleek specimens who were able to reel off the lengths and barely ripple the surface, while I was a classic head-out-of-the-water thrasher, wasting energy and getting nowhere.

Shaw totally altered my swimming style within an hour. By teaching me to look at the bottom of the pool, I released the tension from my neck and shoulders. This helped to stop my body sinking, and I adopted a more horizontal position in the water. Establishing a breathing pattern was harder but, even so, I almost halved the number of strokes it took me to complete a length.

I should then have followed up with Alexander Technique tuition; instead, my next experience was with the co-author of this book. Malcolm Balk took me for a couple of sessions in Regent's Park, where we worked on some of the routines outlined in these pages – particularly those designed to rebalance the relationship between the head and neck and develop appropriate stride patterns and arm movements. My old habits as a jumper and sprinter were still present, especially the tendency to pull my head back and compress the vertebrae in my neck, and what I came to learn was called 'end-gaining': understandable, perhaps, in a sprinter striving for the tape, but unacceptable in someone seeking to run for pleasure and avoid injury.

It was only after these experiences that I took classes at the Westminster Alexander Centre in central London. Here, I struggled to conquer my 'end-gaining' habit and to 'release' over-tensed muscles. But by consciously forestalling my habitual patterns of movement, I learned the importance of keeping my head and back flexible and remaining poised to choose how best to use my body.

These lessons enabled the work of Shaw and Balk to fit into place. They also made intriguing cross-references to some of the other activities I had tried: the sense of release offered in a flotation tank, with the body suspended in an anatomically perfect position; the concentration on the process of movement rather than the end result in Pilates; the precision and balance of tai chi. By a circuitous route, I came to discover how Alexander Technique related to everyday life as well as to sport.

The big four-zero has now come around – which, in athletics terms, qualifies me for veteran status. I have always worked out regularly, including exercise to music classes containing plyometric moves very similar to those I once used in preparation for my flights of triple jump fancy. Competitive instincts still intact, I plan a return to the sport almost two decades after I last set foot on a track. Not to the triple jump, as that would be tempting fate, but to the short sprints and maybe the long jump.

The challenge will be to discover whether youth's raw pace has been replaced by greater self-knowledge. My general running style is now much improved, thanks to the Alexander Technique. We shall see how it holds up when I'm on my blocks, under pressure and staring down the straight…

2. WHAT IS ALEXANDER TECHNIQUE?

Running *aficionados* are well aware that Australia has produced many world record holders, Olympic champions and renowned (if somewhat eccentric) coaches. Athletes like Herb Elliott, Ron Clarke and, more recently, Cathy Freeman, along with such coaches as Percy Cerutty and John Landy, have left an indelible imprint on the history of the sport.

Runners are probably less familiar with another Australian, from northern Tasmania. They might wonder what an actor whose early career was plagued by chronic hoarseness and laryngitis would have to offer a top-class miler, or how his discoveries would influence the training philosophy of a great coach.

Frederick Matthias Alexander specialised in dramatic and humorous monologues. His story reflects a feeling that many runners may have had at one time or another: 'I know I can do better, so why isn't it happening for me? I have all this potential but I don't know how to realise it'. Alexander loved to perform and recite, but he suffered from a problem which prevented him doing so to the best of his ability. Under the rigours of the stage, he would go hoarse to a point where he could not continue and would have to cut his performance short.

Unlike his material, this was no laughing matter. So Alexander did what most of us would have done under the circumstances: he sought help from the medical profession, none of which was very helpful except the advice that he should rest. However, as soon as he put his voice to the test again, the hoarseness would recur.

Finally, after exhausting all available resources, he decided to tackle the problem himself. He reasoned that there must be a link between the way he recited and the difficulty with his voice. To find out what was happening, he set up mirrors so he could observe himself while speaking. He immediately noticed several changes which seemed unnatural: there was an increased tension in his throat, his breathing and his neck as he began to recite. Further observation showed that these changes occurred not just when he spoke, but from the moment he started to think about speaking. 'I saw that as soon as I started to recite, I tended to pull back the head, depress the larynx, and suck in breath through the mouth in such a way as to produce a gasping sound,' he wrote in *The Use of the Self*. He realised that his problem was not just physical, but what he called 'psycho-physical'.

Alexander began to explore different ways to release these tensions. Through experimentation, he discovered that there was a strong inter-connection between his head, neck and back. Any interference with this relationship would not only affect the parts involved, but would affect the rest of what he called 'the self'.

Alexander managed to conquer his hoarseness and was able to project his voice without damaging it. Upon returning to the stage, he encountered other actors with similar problems to his own. He offered them advice and hands-on help, and they would improve as well (Henry Irving, Lillie Langtry and Herbert Beerbohm Tree were among the many actors who later studied what became known as Alexander Technique). He moved to London in 1904, began teaching in New York, and Alexander Technique developed as a way of becoming aware of and preventing the unnecessary tension we put into everything we do, so that we can learn to function in a more free and natural fashion. Alexander continued to take on pupils – he never called them 'patients' – including Aldous Huxley, Adrian Boult and George Bernard Shaw, who started lessons when he was aged 80.

HOW CAN ALEXANDER'S DISCOVERIES HELP RUNNERS?

If Alexander had been a runner rather than an actor, what would his story have been? Perhaps something like this...

As a young man, F. M. (Fast Mother) Alexander was very promising over 800 metres. He enjoyed early success and achieved a national ranking, but was soon plagued by injuries which threatened to end his career. Medical attention, orthotics and a constant supply of gimmicky new shoes provided only short-term relief, because as soon as he resumed serious training he would injure himself once again and be forced back into the tedious process of rest and rehab.

When doctors proposed risky surgery as the only solution, Alexander decided to take matters into his own hands. He reasoned that there must be something in the way he ran that was causing his problems, since he only got injured when he trained hard and raced. Setting up a video camera, he filmed himself from several angles. It was only on viewing the results that he noticed several things his track pals had often joked about. When he ran, he tended to pull his head back, breathe in loudly through his mouth, tighten and arch his lower back, and pound his feet on the ground. His friends told him that these habits were more pronounced at the finish of a race, when he looked like someone who was being attacked by a swarm of bees. Further study revealed that many of these running habits were also present when he walked, though then they were less noticeable.

Through constant observation and experimentation, Alexander found that if he could maintain the poise of his head on top of his spine when he ran, this had a positive influence on the rest of his body patterns: he stopped gasping for air, arching and stiffening his back, and the ground no longer echoed to the pounding of his feet.

However, maintaining these improvements when he ran and particularly when he raced proved more difficult. He noticed that he would usually revert to his old habits in moments of pressure or stress...

See the similarities? Let's look at how Alexander's discoveries could help his middle distance-running namesake.

ALEXANDER'S DISCOVERIES

F. M. Alexander was neither a runner nor a coach, although, like most Aussies, he maintained a keen interest in sport. Did he work specifically with athletes? No again, although in one of his books he did offer some constructive comments on the unfortunate finish of Dorando Pietri in the 1908 Olympic marathon – he collapsed within sight of the tape and had to be helped across the line. However, running and reciting have one key thing in common: what Alexander called 'use of the self'. Acts can be performed in a number of ways, some of which are less harmful than others. The implication is that the way we are doing it will have an influence on the outcome; or, to quote the man himself, 'the way you use yourself affects the way you function'.

Let's employ a mechanical metaphor to make the point clear. As a runner, you are both car *and* driver. You only get one vehicle in this life, and in spite of advances in replacement technology (new hips, knee reconstructions), the

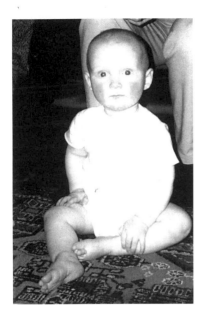

Small children usually demonstrate excellent 'primary control of use'.

original parts generally work best. So if you blow the engine, strip the tyres, fry the brakes and stain the upholstery, you can't trade it in for a new model. As driving instructors everywhere will tell you, we all bring attitudes, skills and habits to bear on the way our car performs on the road. We pop the clutch, slam on the brakes, over-rev the engine, reverse into bollards and fail to look in the mirror before changing lanes. All these factors contribute to the functioning of the vehicle and, ultimately, the quality of the ride.

● **Primary control of use.** Alexander found that his voice difficulties were related to a pattern of interference in the natural relationship between his head, neck and back, which was linked to the way he used his whole organism in the act of reciting. He realised that his head-neck-back relationship was the key area to focus on when 'unlearning' the body's habitual reactions and tensions, and called it the primary control of use. This relationship exerts a powerful influence on the way we function (including, of course, the way we run). It can be described in its ideal form as the state which is achieved when the neck is free of tension, and the head is therefore not pulled down into the spine: ease, effortlessness and a sense of lightness in movement. The head is poised freely on top of the spine in such a way that the spine is encouraged to lengthen and the back to widen. In other words, what coaches describe as 'running tall'.

When Sebastian Coe set a new 800 metres world record of 1 min 42.4 secs, taking a second off Alberto Juantorena's previous best, he said of his performance: 'I had no sensation of speed and I think I could have run even faster…it was a strange feeling, like being on auto pilot; I was mentally outside what my body was achieving and it just felt beautiful'. This state of flow, often described as being 'in the zone' or 'peak experience', is spoken of in near-mystical, Zen-like terms. Athletes often resort to various rituals in the hope of maintaining or rediscovering that elusive 'state of grace'.

Professor V. Abrahams of Queens University in Canada, a leading medical researcher on neck muscles and their importance, insists: 'The evidence that the neck plays a critical role in posture is overwhelming'. In an experiment designed to demonstrate this fact, a volunteer had a local anaesthetic injected into one side of his neck. The loss of muscle sensation and of muscle tone on the injected side gave an illusion of falling over to that side. The subject reported that he felt drawn to one side like an iron bar to a magnet. He was unable to walk with any co-ordination, like someone who has had too much to drink. When lying down, he felt the couch was toppling over towards the side of the injection. As David Garlick points out in *The Lost Sixth Sense*: 'The dominating nerve inputs from the neck help to determine how the brain controls muscles in posture and movement'.

Alexander spent a considerable amount of time observing himself in the mirror – not unlike many actors today, no doubt. However, Alexander's purpose was not to check for signs of a receding hairline, but to discover why his voice seemed to disappear, especially when he needed it most – on stage. While he watched himself recite in the mirror, he did several peculiar things which he surmised were related to his vocal difficulties. They included tightening his neck and lifting his chin so that his head was pulled back, depressing his larynx and breathing in through his mouth with a loud gasping sound. He subsequently noticed that he also lifted his chest, arched his back and tightened his legs and feet. What a mess…

As Alexander remarked in his third book, *The Use of the Self*: 'Where was I to begin? Was it the sucking in of breath that caused the pulling back of the head and the depressing of the larynx?' What he found was that he could not change his breathing or the contraction of his larynx directly, but he could control these harmful tendencies *indirectly* by preventing his head from being pulled back. Further research enabled him to see that the relationship between his head and neck also affected his torso; and for his voice to be allowed to work properly, his head had to be carried in such a way as to encourage his back to lengthen and widen.

Phew, you say, this is getting pretty complicated. Not so. Try this:

Sit on a chair, near the edge, and allow yourself to slump. Feels great, right? But you might notice that the back of your neck has 'disappeared' and your throat feels a little tight. This is related to what Alexander was talking about. Now sit up really straight, so that your chest is raised, your back is hollowed and your chin is tucked in. You may notice the same feeling in your throat – which was, after all, Alexander's focus. This is the sort of thing he tried to do when correcting the way he carried his head.

Our co-ordination is affected by the quality of the relationship between the head, neck and back. When we over-contract the neck and pull the head down, the spine compresses and distorts – which affects the way we use our limbs. It then takes more effort to get from A to B, and we place more strain on ourselves in the process. In other words, someone like this will tend to run 'a bit funny' and not make the best use of themselves. A bit like trying to push a rope up a hill: it can be done, but…

Vertebrate animals generally demonstrate good co-ordination: their head leads and their body follows. Of course, animals do not *know* what they are doing, they 'just do it'. We humans, on the other hand, have the mixed blessing of consciousness, which can be used to help us become a bit more cheetah-like in our urban jungle.

People from less industrialised nations seem to suffer less interference with the natural use of themselves than we do in the west. For example, physiologists have found that a Kenyan woman uses no more effort – that is, oxygen consumption – walking up a hill with a 10kg jug of water balanced on her head than you or I without one. And, as far as I know, they haven't yet figured out why.

It is probably because Kenyan women already possess excellent balance and co-ordination. You don't see Kenyan men walking around with jugs balanced on their heads, but you certainly see enough of them on the winners' rostrum at races.

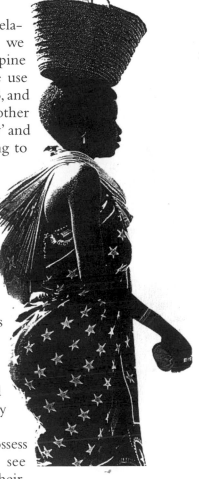

Ease, balance and co-ordination in motion.

● **Faulty sensory awareness** was how Alexander described one of the most important and basic factors underlying habitual misuse patterns in the way we do things. It refers to the way that we think or feel we are doing one thing when in fact we are doing something completely different. People who see themselves on video or in photographs are often surprised to see what they *really* look like. This is important when we try to change an ingrained habit.

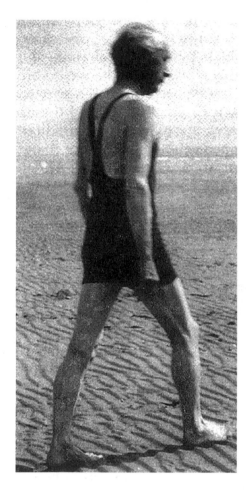

Even in old age, F. M. Alexander continued to show poise and a beautifully lengthened back.

The new and improved version often feels odd, awkward or even wrong – which increases the likelihood of going back to what we know, even if it isn't serving us well.

As a runner, you might find yourself in the following dilemma. You've just read an article on improving your running form and have decided to heed its suggestions. This decision was prompted in part by a recent picture of yourself in action looking more like a Skoda with four flat tyres than a Jaguar purring along at full throttle. And there was also that injudicious comment by a fellow athlete who said she could recognise you, even at a distance, because of the cute way you roll your shoulders and hold your head on one side – not to mention that little hitch in your stride. After several weeks of visualising running like a puppet and doing appropriate exercises, you are starting to believe that real progress is being made.

Much to your dismay, after videoing yourself to preserve the new you for posterity, you are shocked to see that the cute way you cock your head and roll your shoulders is still there. In fact, it seems worse! You feel upset and let down. You ask: 'How could my senses have deceived me?'

Alexander offered a clue when he remarked that: 'You can't know a thing by an instrument that is wrong'. The instrument to which he was referring was our *kinaesthetic sense* – our ability to know where one bit of our body is in relation to another, either at rest or in movement. The difficulty Alexander encountered, and which is widespread in today's society, he called faulty sensory awareness: the inability of our kinaesthetic sense to provide an accurate picture of what we are doing with ourselves – in this case, how we are running. The familiar becomes the standard by which we judge what is right and what is wrong. Since the runner in our scenario was trying hard to improve, we can guess with some certainty that s/he was doing what *felt right* – that is, rolling the shoulders and tilting the head. The challenge when trying to change an old habit is to become comfortable with the unfamiliar: something which is difficult to do under the best of circumstances, but particularly hard when one is striving to 'get it right'. 'Trying,' Alexander said, 'only emphasises what we know already.'

Chronic tension also plays a role in faulty sensory awareness. Muscles which are tightened for any period of time no longer provide the brain with feedback. In other words, we are no longer aware of what is going on in these areas, and it becomes harder to make the decisions necessary to maintain our pace, health or enjoyment.

A 1992 study looked at the advantages and disadvantages of running when 'associated' (switched-on) and 'disassociated' (switched-off). People who disassociate tend to distract themselves from discomfort, pain or tedium by thinking of something more pleasant – for example, a warm beach (how many people, when sloshing through the icy winter rain, have not imagined themselves by the water's edge, catching the rays?). But runners who associate, the research showed, pay more attention to the signals coming from their muscles, and use this information to release build-ups of tension. In the study, the latter group performed better. This suggests that runners benefit from paying attention, and relaying accurate information to the brain.

There are other disadvantages to what Professor Frank Pierce Jones, one of the first teachers to conduct scientific research on the Alexander Technique, called 'automatic performance'. The chief of these is that without awareness, things cannot be changed. Socrates, when asked whether it was better to do wrong knowingly or unknowingly, shocked his listeners by replying that it was better to do wrong knowingly. If you know that it is wrong, he explained, you can change.

A wonderful example of the joys of faulty sensory awareness appeared in an article by Geoffrey Cannon in the November 1987 issue of *Running Times*:

'I've never been the same,' he wrote, 'since a run round Hyde Park and Kensington Gardens in newly fallen snow, early one winter morning four years ago. I was scheduled for three circuits: thirteen-and-a-half miles at a steady eight-minute-mile pace, making 1 hr 48 mins for the whole run. No big deal,

I thought, and eased into the run feeling pretty pleased with myself. Nobody else was around. Or so I thought, until I reached Speakers' Corner. For there, by my side, on my own route, were a runner's footprints – and a funny sight they were, too. The prints were man-size, but the runner was taking comic little strides. What was sillier still, though, was the position of the footprints. They looked like a clock showing five minutes to two: the left foot splayed out a bit, the right foot turned some way to being back to front. A fine figure of fun he must look, I thought to myself smugly, and carried on. Doesn't he realise how ridiculous he looks? I amused myself around Hyde Park Corner by imitating the gait of the stumbler who, no doubt, I should soon ease past.

'I never saw him, though. Instead, I was startled to see, the next time round Speakers' Corner, that there were two sets of footprints, one fairly crisp, the other half-obscured by falling snow, right by my side, on my route. Surely there couldn't be two runners, I thought to myself. It had to be one. Odd, that I hadn't caught him up. So I amused myself by running in his footprints.

'And then I realised. He was me. I had no idea I ran like that. For the rest of the run I tried not to believe my eyes. This must stop, I instructed myself, and made my feet parallel, and ran round in little circles to check myself out. And still the feet – my feet – were not straight. I finished the run completely deflated.

'A few weeks later I could bear it no longer, and decided to have a confidential word with a compassionate runner. So I asked my co-author Alison Turnbull: "Ali, do I ever run like this?" (deliberately exaggerating the lop-sided duck's gait). "All the time," she said. "I can tell it's you 200 yards away." And she pointed out some hilarious little ways I have with my arms when I run. I was forced to admit that, like so many runners, I had a completely inaccurate mental picture of myself in action.

'Only then did I notice that the "Permanent Record Of You To Treasure Always" photographs taken in New York's Central Park at the end of the marathon showed the real picture; as did reflective shop windows into which I started nervously glancing. Hence my interest in movement awareness in general, and Alexander Technique in particular…'

● **Recognition of the force of habit** is another central tenet of Alexander Technique. The price of freedom, so the saying goes, is eternal vigilance. But anyone who has ever tried to change a deeply ingrained habit knows how easy it is to slip back into the old patterns. This seems to be particularly true where runners are concerned!

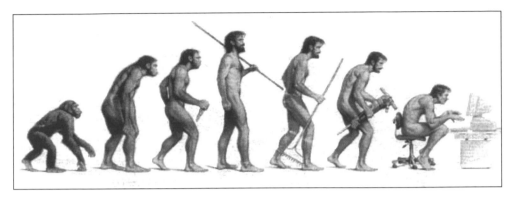

'Somewhere, something went terribly wrong.'

We've all heard of those addicts (and there is no better word to describe them) who simply have to get their training run in, no matter weather conditions, illness, injury, time of day (or night) – and for no good reason other than to record the mileage in their meticulously-maintained diaries. I once trained with someone who was so obsessed with keeping an accurate record of his efforts that when he cracked his head painfully on a low branch, almost knocking himself out, he still managed to stop his watch before hitting the ground!

The bad news is that this kind of behaviour can lead to problems in life as a whole, not to mention poorer performance due to over-training. The good news is that the same qualities of persistence and determination, when expressed in a more balanced way, are exactly what are required to conquer bad habits and achieve a higher level of functioning.

I think it is important to mention the difference between habits which are developed consciously and those which sneaked in when we weren't looking. To go back to the car/driver analogy; you may have learned to drive by following a series of steps, such as: get in, put on seat belt, put key in ignition, and so on. With experience, you can follow these steps in a state close to unconsciousness, as many of us do on early mornings on the way to work. But, and this is the difference, if you ever found yourself in a different make of car with which you were not familiar, you could, by reviewing the basics, probably figure out how to drive it. If you never went through the process of learning the basics, it would be more difficult. Consciously learned habits are easier to change.

My story – Roy

I started long-distance running in my late teens, and over the next five years completed a number of marathons, half-marathons and ten-mile races. I suffered minor aches and pains, but assumed they were normal for a runner and continued to race. When I began to experience problems with my back, I consulted my doctor who advised me to stop and prevent further complications.

Reluctantly I followed his recommendation and looked to other sports to fill the gap. However, the back pain gradually increased to a point where it affected my work and restricted my sporting activities. Treatment from physiotherapists, osteopaths and chiropractors gave only a few days' relief from the pain. As a last resort I went for Alexander Technique lessons and was so impressed that I enrolled to train as a teacher myself.

During my training I went on one of Malcolm Balk's courses and found there was an easier and more efficient way of running. With guidance from Malcolm, you can learn how to overcome your habitual movements and allow the reflexes to perform their function as nature intended – it's like taking your foot off the brake and running on air. However, because old habits do not go away that easily, it does take time and constant awareness to be able to maintain. Over the next four years I continued to attend Malcolm's courses and was able to step up my running schedule at no cost to my health.

Looking back at my old finishing-line photographs, I can now appreciate what had contributed to my problems. The most noticeable was the tendency to pull my knees inwards as I ran, while my feet landed with the toes pointing out – causing the knee to collapse in further as I pushed off from the ground. I twisted the upper torso and held my arms by my side, giving the impression that I was moving in different directions – the lower half in a linear fashion, while the upper had a lateral motion effectively cutting my body in two.

I had never given much thought to how I actually ran, so this action felt normal. When I first started to apply the Alexander Technique, it felt very different and awkward. After many years spent running with my own particular style, any changes would inevitably feel wrong. Yet, as my old habitual technique had been the cause of numerous injuries, it was obviously not the most efficient. I reasoned that if it felt wrong, then I must have been moving in the right direction away from my previously poor technique.

To overcome my habit of pulling in the knees, I would think of them moving outward. This initially felt like running with a bow-leg action, although as pulling them in had always seemed normal this was to be expected. An awareness of the hip, knee and ankle joints enabled a more natural swing of the leg, promoting a springier step with better shock absorption. By using my arms, I started to run with the sense of my whole self being involved with the action and not just the legs. With practice, my self-awareness increased to a point where I could identify areas of excessive muscular tension or where I was putting in too much effort to run. My neck and shoulders released, I stopped holding my torso, allowing my breathing to open up. And my legs began to swing from the hip, thus removing the twist.

I appreciate that this will be a continuous process. But I now have a new approach to running that has made it a joy, where previously this was not always the case. I don't really give much thought to my times, but the distances are gradually increasing with no recurrence of old injuries.

Running, after all, is a natural, symmetrical activity that can be a lot easier if we learn to stop doing the things that interfere with the movement. Habit is one of the most fundamental factors of performance, but because we are unaware of its influence it tends to be ignored at our expense.

● **Inhibition and direction.** These are technical terms which refer to essential processes of Alexander Technique. 'Inhibition' is a decision not to react immediately to a stimulus. 'Direction' involves projecting conscious intentions to oneself without actually doing them. 'Directions' in Alexander Technique are essentially preventive thoughts – that is, thinking to stop what you don't want to occur rather than positively getting something to happen. These, therefore, are skills that can help a runner eliminate and prevent what is not necessary, and encourage and maintain what needs to take place.

A runner I once coached at 800 metres and 1,500 metres decided to give the marathon a try. A friend offered him the following advice, which provides a perfect illustration of 'inhibition'. He said: 'Ian, the first time you feel like going [that is, increasing your pace], *don't!* The second time you feel like going, *don't!!* The third time you feel like going, if you still have something left, *go!!!*'. The good news is that in his first marathon, Ian, a talented middle-distancer weighing 83 kg (13 st 3 lbs), ran five minutes faster than his objective to finish in a very respectable 2 hr 31 mins.

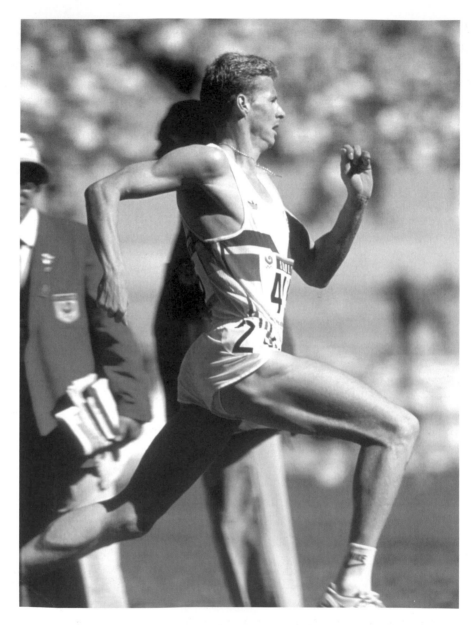

Steve Cram competing in the 1,500 metres at the 1988 Seoul Olympics: running at this level requires the athlete to 'think in activity' and employ choice rather than mere habit.

Alexander originally developed the skill which he called 'inhibition' to help him change a pattern which was threatening his career. He had to re-learn how to recite without putting so much strain on his vocal apparatus that it would fail him when he needed it most – when he was on stage, alone, trying to entertain the crowd. Inhibition was the key that eventually enabled him to improve not only his voice, but his overall health.

Simply put, inhibition is a matter of taking advantage of the space between stimulus and response, between when you decide to do something and the moment you put that decision into action. We could formalise this as follows:

Stimulus: increase speed.
Pause (inhibition): prevent tendency to tighten back of the neck, lift shoulders, push head forward, and so on.
Direction: think about where you want your arms to travel if you were to increase their rhythm.
Response: let it happen (that is, release into it happening rather than contract).

Untying our responses from the stimuli that provoke them can open up all kinds of possibilities. Old habits can be eliminated and new ones explored and cultivated. It's a bit like driving the car with the handbrake on: even if you're going in the right direction, there is still some resistance.

Learning to inhibit the old, unwanted response permits the new to occur unimpeded. And inhibition is a skill we need to survive: remembering to pause and look both ways at a road junction can do much to prolong a running career! The challenge is remembering to remember.

I used to tell my pupils that the first stage of learning Alexander Technique was awareness. I don't believe that is true for many people because, for awareness to be of any use, it needs to be there before we act. Thinking 'Whoops! I should have looked before crossing the street' as the truck drives over your toes makes this point painfully clear.

Alexander said that we need to wake up, to quicken the mind. A simple task I give my pupils is to ask them to pause before standing up, even if it's only for one second. They often report back that they had stood up and were halfway out of the room before they remembered, if they remembered at all. I have a hard time trying to get sprinters to pause before tackling an acceleration so that they have time to review certain technical demands. By the time they're running, it's too late: they have to pause and think (what Alexander called 'direct') before they act. As Alexander found with reciting, just the idea is enough to cause a habitual reaction.

● **Non-doing**. Another Alexander technical term, it certainly does not mean doing nothing! 'Non-doing' implies two things when you carry out an action: first, refrain from over-employing parts of yourself that you don't need in the action (for example, moving the arms does not necessarily mean you have to lift the shoulders as well). Second, allow joints to 'undo' when moving and refrain from clamping joint surfaces against each other. Alexander highlighted the importance of using an appropriate amount of effort for the task in hand. Hence the idea of 'less is more' – as long as it's the right kind of less!

ANATOMY OF AN ALEXANDER TECHNIQUE LESSON – FRED

Fred is a 53-year-old professional man in good shape, who has taken six Alexander Technique lessons. He has been trying to run ten kilometres in under 40 minutes for the past three years. In order to achieve this goal, he paid for a training programme designed to help him reach his target in 12 weeks…

Although the programme seemed straight forward and do-able, Fred was not able to manage it. He found he could not complete the workouts, even though they were within his range. While it might have been useful to analyse the programme itself for inherent strengths and weaknesses, merely watching Fred run revealed problems which were blocking his potential, increasing the stress levels of his activity and making his training much harder than it needed to be.

Fred was not very 'connected' or aware of how he ran. He leant his head to one side, pushed his pelvis into his legs and crossed one leg in front of the other on each stride. His body wobbled, he looked down and frowned, while his shoulders were held in an elevated position. It seemed that he was trying too hard to get it right, and was thinking in terms of results rather than the process needed to achieve them. As a consequence, his attention would wander.

The challenge was to get Fred to slow down enough so that he could begin to 'think in activity'. Why? So that his running would be more determined by choice (conscious) than habit (unconscious), thus helping him to reduce or eliminate the tics and improve his performance and enjoyment.

We began the lesson with some table work, with Fred lying on his back, head raised a little on a small pile of books, and his feet drawn up near him so his knees were bent. While Fred was lying down, we worked to reduce the interference with the head-neck-back pattern and to help him begin to get a sense of lengthening.

Once this had been established, I asked Fred to think of lifting an arm – first explaining that if the shoulder joint was free, the arm could move independently from the torso. If his shoulder was fixed, lifting the arm would cause his back to move or his neck to stiffen. I asked him to notice if anything like this occurred during the movement. His response to this suggestion was instantaneous: he immediately lifted his arm then dropped it back down to the table. During this procedure, it was apparent that Fred's head was lolling to one side, he was frowning with concentration, and was clearly in a hurry to get on with it! He moved his arms one after the other, then announced, somewhat triumphantly, that he'd noticed nothing.

I then explained that the hip joint was likewise designed to allow his leg to move independently from his back. I asked him to renew his intention to lengthen, lift his leg off the table, straighten it out and let it rest again, and see what changed. This time he noticed that his pelvis rolled to one side and that he tightened his stomach muscles. There were a few other 'adjustments' which he was not aware of, such as the frowning and holding his head on one side. What's more, he had focused all his attention on his leg and had forgotten about what was going on elsewhere.

I got Fred off the table and we did a little work standing. As he began to become aware of what he was doing while standing, Fred noticed his tendency to hyper-extend his knees and arch his lower back – or, as he put it, assume the 'piss position'! We then worked on maintaining his length while beginning to allow his legs to release and his lower back to 'fill out' (widen). This took the pressure off his lower back and also helped to free up his ribs so that he was able to breathe more easily.

Before beginning to run, I asked Fred to treat this as a learning experience and not as a training session, in that I would stop him frequently to explain, ask for feedback, re-establish conscious directional instructions, release tension, and so on. This was important, as he might have become even more upset at not being able to run as he was used to. Furthermore, many runners consider stopping as a form of cheating, or at least a sign of weakness: 'Real runners never walk…'

Outside, I had him renew his preventive directions for the head-neck-back and for his legs, especially to free up the front of the ankles and the back of his knees in order to create the right conditions for uninhibited movement. Once this was established, I asked him where he tended to focus his gaze. Fred spotted fairly quickly that he would usually look down at the ground about a metre in front of him, and that his head followed his eyes, tilting forward from the base of the neck.

When I asked him to think about 'aiming higher', he noticed that he was a little lighter on his feet but that the urge to look down was extremely powerful and that he could only maintain his long view for a few seconds before needing to look down again. I asked Fred simply to be aware of what was happening, and to give preventive directions to himself: 'think up rather than down', 'eyes looking out rather than to the ground', and so on. I helped him in this awakening process by drawing his attention to what was going on, as well as maintaining a light hand on his neck which helped to renew his length.

This process served several purposes. First, giving preventive directions enabled him to be more aware of how he tended to misuse himself – in Fred's case, dropping his head from the base of his neck, and stiffening his ankles and knees. Second, the directions prepared the releases needed literally to allow the next step. Third, the directions helped to maintain the conditions for free and efficient movement – freeing the back of the knees (that is, refusing to stiffen them) allowed his knees to bend more easily, with less interference.

BENEFITS OF ALEXANDER TECHNIQUE FOR RUNNERS

● **Universality.** Alexander Technique can be applied anywhere, any time. It requires no special equipment or help. It can and should be used before, during and after running.

● **Autonomy.** Like a language, once you learn Alexander Technique and how to apply it, you don't have depend on someone else – whose title usually ends in *-practor* or *-path* – to benefit from it. It's yours to do with as you wish.

● **It deals with causes, not just symptoms.** As a result, people who learn Alexander Technique often benefit in many areas of their lives as part of a generalised, ongoing process of improvement.

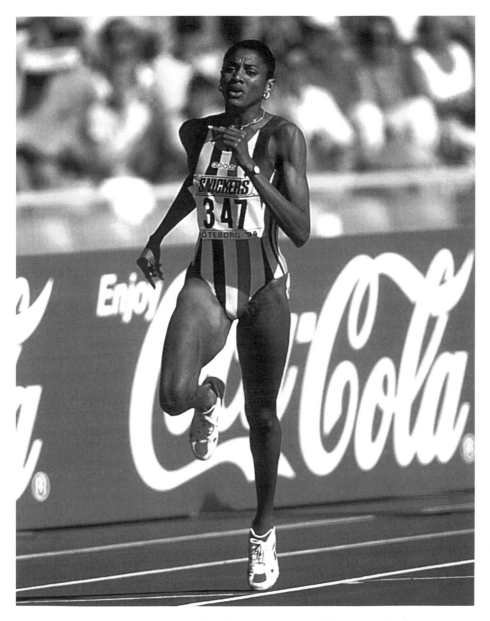

Marie-Jose Perec winning gold at the 1995 World Championships:
a great illustration of 'running tall'.

●**You can get more with less.** Improvements in balance and co-ordination lead to more efficient movement with less wasted effort. Energy can be directed to where it will give the greatest return.

● **Injury prevention.** Tuning in to the feedback and signals enables the runner to back off before the 'niggle becomes a nightmare'.

● **Development of fitness and form.** The late George Sheehan, doctor, runner, writer and philosopher, wrote this when in his 70s: 'One way I have aged is in my appearance and in the way I go about normal activities. Carriage is important – and mine is poor. Having good posture, flexibility and a spring in your step makes for a youthful impression. But I have poor flexibility, terrible posture, and tend to stroll rather than stride. If you saw me walking around town, you would think I was older than I am. This form of ageing is, of course, completely unnecessary!!' (my exclamations)

Often in trying to reach our goals, we sacrifice form for fitness. This is a mistake, and results in unnecessary stress and strain which ultimately work against the original intention. I can remember back to my days as an ice hockey player, when in innocent arrogance I believed that my abilities and success were clear indications of my highly developed co-ordination and evolution as a human being. The fact that my 'form' was really pathetic the moment I got off the ice was of little concern to me up to this point. In fact, I used to revel in my version of 'cat-like' repose – for which, read 'collapse'.

It was only when my superior beliefs about my co-ordination were put to the test as I tried to apply my habitual approach to playing the cello, that I began to suspect all was not as wonderful as I might have believed. At the cello, I was stiff and my attitude decreased my ability to learn. It was only when I began taking Alexander Technique lessons that the blinkers really came off. I was increasingly aware of my tendency to slump and collapse (like many athletes, dancers and musicians who stop 'thinking' once they finish performing). It was as if I was disconnecting from my body.

Another area for scrutiny was my tendency, when things weren't going well, to force, to push, to seek a 'bigger hammer'. Looking back, it is funny how this 'attitude' is not something that simply manifested itself physically but was present in all areas of life. You might well imagine the problems of adjustment I had to the British way of doing things – ways which, as a North American, I found incredibly slow and senseless (the joy of cashing a cheque, for example).

The basic message here is that if a runner sacrifices form for fitness, trouble is usually not far off. Training when injured or sick is an example of putting 'fitness' before 'form' (that is, common sense and health).

● **Recuperation and regeneration.** The ironic thing about running or any other form of endurance activity is that the improvements occur mostly when we stop – that is, when our bodies are compensating for the stress to which they have been subjected. This is known as the training effect. In many ways, knowing how and when to stop becomes as important as knowing how and when to train.

Countless runners have lost the potential benefits of a training programme by not giving themselves enough time to recover, and risking the dangers of over-training or even burnout. As a coach, I strongly encourage my athletes to take at least one day a week of complete rest. However, it can be very difficult to persuade highly-motivated athletes (super-'end-gainers') that less (training) will actually be more in terms of fitness. 'End-gaining' is a term Alexander used to refer to our urgency to reach our goals too quickly, without due consideration of the means whereby we might achieve them easily and without harm.

On another level, the 'active rest' attitude taught as part of the Technique is an extremely effective means of 'getting yourself sorted'. In other words, rather than collapsing in front of the TV, the runner can use the active rest procedure to release any unnecessary tension and re-establish a state of balanced co-ordination which will go a long way towards helping them reap the benefits of the training regime.

● **Improvement.** It is sad but true that most people who take up running never learn to run well. This is not just true of runners: a quick trip to your local tennis court or golf course will give you innumerable examples of people playing poorly. There are many reasons for this, two of which we discuss at length in this book: end-gaining and faulty sensory awareness. Like a variation on an old joke, 90 per cent of runners are confirmed end-gainers, while the other ten per cent are confirmed liars!

While goals can provide an important source of motivation for runners, focusing too quickly on them can be a case of putting the cart before the horse: 'I must finish that 10k in under 45 mins', or 'I have to run a marathon', and the list goes on and on. Runners, especially at the early stage of their careers, are vulnerable to developing bad habits of form which will plague them for their entire running lives. On the other hand, the running Alexandrian will take the time needed to learn to run well. I estimate that it takes a person of average co-ordination who wants to run competitively around five years.

Fred, the runner in the Alexander lesson illustration, 'ran heavy' – you could really hear him coming. But when Fred applied the principles he had learned, such as maintaining his intention through inhibition (noticing when his mind wandered and refocusing), and direction (reminding himself not to look down), he could modify it and run much more lightly. The only problem was that he kept forgetting to pay attention and would quickly lapse into his old pattern of pounding. Finally, after I had brought his attention back to this habit once again, he exclaimed in exasperation: 'How bloody often do I have think about my bloody feet landing?' And of course the answer was: 'Every bloody step!'

Alexandrians will smile at this story, for it may reflect some of their own struggles in learning to pay attention. Now this is not as ominous a task as it may seem. Back to the car: when you learn to drive, at first you have to think about putting the key in the ignition, turning it on, and so on. Once you become more familiar with the basics, you don't have to think about them so actively – but at the same time, in order to move the vehicle, *you can't leave any of them out*. Learning to 'think in activity', as John Dewey once described Alexander Technique, is a skill which can help a runner improve.

● **Choice.** There are many different ways of running: fast, slow, uphill or down, into the wind, on different surfaces, in hot or cold weather, with a side stitch, at various altitudes, straight, zig-zaggy, alone or in a pack, on the track, on the beach. You get the idea. Good runners adapt their running form in order to meet each condition effectively. Variations in form include lengthening or shortening the stride, more or less use of the arms, changing the amount of forward lean, the amount of knee or heel lift, landing more towards the heel or more towards the ball of the foot, varying breathing rhythms, and so on. Poor running form, and lack of awareness of both oneself and one's environ-ment, lead to statements like: 'I can't run fast/uphill/downhill when it's cold.' Chosing not to run outside when it's minus-30 degrees and you are worried about frostbite can be a wise decision, but not running outside at all in the winter because you don't know how to do it safely is denying yourself a poten-tially wonderful experience.

Alexandrians find that developing their overall balance, co-ordination and awareness puts more tools in their belt and allows them to adapt to the circumstances at hand.

● **Enjoyment.** You can take pleasure in performing the art of running well, whatever that means to you. It might be running slowly yet lightly and elegantly through a park near your home. It might be floating rather than pounding on the treadmill at the gym, your body staying quiet and poised as your arms move rhythmically in synch with your legs. It might be finding that extra gear on the home straight and maintaining your form to the finish line. Or climbing a long hill with effortless ease, your body finding the perfect angle as you lean gently into the slope, your knees popping up with every stride and your arm movement helping to keep you light and tall over the crest.

The runner who learns to practise the art of running with an Alexandrian attitude will experience many such moments.

My Story – Juliet

I do not consider myself to be a serious runner or sportswoman. Yet I really enjoy running. It keeps me fit, and I like to experience the movement of my body. I run about once a week, in green open spaces if possible.

There are certain things I have noticed about being a female runner. One is my desire to be as good as the men, which leads to me pushing myself in a rigid way. The other is a need to avoid attracting attention. This seems inevitable when I'm running alone, therefore I try to make myself invisible. However, I want to describe the times when I have managed to free myself from habits which restrict me in both these situations.

Before I started having regular Alexander Technique lessons and began training to become a teacher, I always felt as if I was running against myself. My 'use' was not good – I had a strong pattern of hunching my shoulders up, pulling my head back, pushing my hips forward and bracing myself against whatever I happened to be doing. I thought exercise would be good for me, but with a back problem and this particular way of using my body, I don't think it was.

This has all started to change as I have explored the Technique. I continued to run regularly while training to become an Alexander Technique teacher, and had occasional running lessons with Malcolm Balk. This shed light on my approach to exercise, which was one of 'no pain, no gain'. Somehow, I felt that because I only managed to run once a week I'd better make the most of it. So I'd let the desire to do an extra lap of the park outweigh the pleasure of the moment, and push myself when I was already tired. It is one thing gently to challenge one's limitations and go just a bit further; quite another to tighten up, grit one's teeth and force it. This is when I could feel my body stiffening up. Old habits would kick in, as if I was holding myself together until I got to the end.

One particular habit was to tense the muscles of my torso so my breathing would become constricted. Another was to look at the ground, causing my upper body to pull down and leading to a drawing in and hunching of my

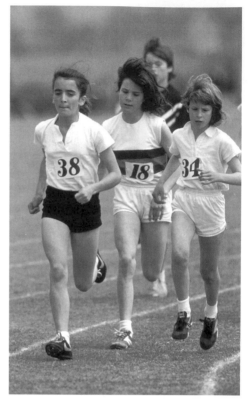

Young girls often demonstrate excellent form: their challenge is to 'run tall' and avoid pulling down as greater self-consciousness develops in their teens.

shoulders. There were two reasons for doing this: the first, purely practical – to keep an eye out for loose paving stones and avoid the ubiquitous dog poo! The other stemmed from a self-consciousness about running in public.

When I'm out, I don't see many other women running. Those that are usually run with someone else. I mostly see men running alone, doing so with a certain confidence. In contrast, I feel conspicuous and imagine that I'm on show. I think it is a fact of life that women are out on the streets at night less often than men, and the same goes for running – even in the daytime. My impression is that women are drawn more to exercising indoors, in groups. So I'm aware that as a young woman running alone around the neighbourhood or in the park, men look at me. In my efforts to become invisible I have tended to look down, hoping that I'll be noticed less.

However, this looking down just pulls me down further. I have learned to counteract the habit, to look up and around me as I run, as well as keeping a peripheral eye on the ground. This has helped me to feel more confident about being out there, doing my own thing. As a result, my technique has improved: looking up helps me to stay back and up, so that I can release more easily in my neck and shoulders and move in a lighter way.

These habits, of wanting both to push until the end and to keep myself invisible, have changed over time. I had one experience when I was able to turn them around in a few powerful moments. Surprisingly, it was at the end of a run, and I was looking down, pulling down, my legs were tight and my shoulders were moving towards my ears in a painfully familiar way.

I was tired. But then I suddenly thought, 'I don't need to be like this'. I said to myself, 'Look up, stay back and up'. I felt a strong release of energy as the instructions took effect: everything which had been dragging me down uncoiled in an instant. I really was going up. I kept going past my house, where I had intended to stop, and around the neighbourhood saying to myself, 'I'll just go as far as that tree and stop'. But when I got to the tree I didn't want to stop. I kept on finding new markers. This went on for about 15 minutes. When I did finally stop, it was because I didn't want to overdo it rather than because I was particularly tired. It was the longest run I'd done for some time, but it wasn't the length that made it significant – it was the knowledge that I could break out of bad habits. It was hugely encouraging to discover that I could change the way I work with my body and mind.

Then I made another discovery: that I was able to run downhill. This might not sound particularly clever, but it was exciting for me. I was in Wales with my friend Karen, and we had climbed to the top of a ridge in the Brecon Beacons. We were sheltered by a higher ridge on one side, and on the other we looked down over the valley. Houses and barns were scattered around, while green patches of forest clustered near a reservoir. It was early spring, everything looked delightfully golden, and the weather was fresh and windy. I felt relaxed with so much clean air in my lungs, and deeply at ease. There was no-one else in sight.

We had been so engaged in conversation that we had forgotten the time, and realised that we had to get back to where we were staying pretty quickly. We started walking down the hillside, but then I said to Karen, 'Why not run?' I was wearing sturdy boots and just relaxed as I started to let gravity take me downwards, gradually speeding up the movement. I remembered what I had learned about not resisting the slope – staying back and up at the same time as going with the gradient. Every time I felt myself wanting to brace back or tighten from fear of falling, I just relaxed, kept concentrating on where I was putting my feet (the ground wasn't particularly even), and looked up. I let my hips soften and released my legs while working to keep my feet firmly in contact with the ground each time they landed. It was exhilarating – I felt so free.

Karen had been struggling to keep up with me, but I had been shouting out tips which I hoped would help her to relax. She said, once we reached the bottom, that initially she was terrified, then she followed my pointers and saw that I wasn't falling over which helped her to realise it could work. And she did get there with me.

It goes without saying that I need continually to work with these old habits, to give myself directions and keep aware of myself and my surroundings whenever I run or walk. The Alexander Technique does not offer a magical cure: I must always engage my attention and put in the effort. But I know that the tools I have gained will keep me alive to the sheer beauty of movement.

3. WHAT IS FITNESS?

Good question! Fitness is a word with different meanings. In a purely physical sense, fitness is the ability of the heart, lungs and muscles to function at optimal efficiency. However, the definition of fitness is widening. As Rodney Cullum and the late Lesley Mowbray explain in *The YMCA Guide to Exercise to Music*: 'Total fitness includes physical, nutritional, medical, mental, emotional and social fitness. It can be described as the ability to meet the demands of the environment, plus a little in reserve for emergencies'.
The more restricted definition divides fitness into five basic components:

• Cardio-vascular fitness, otherwise known as stamina, endurance or aerobic fitness. This is the efficiency of the heart, lungs and circulatory system.

• Muscular strength, or the ability of a muscle to exert maximum force to overcome a resistance. By increasing the amount of resistance, the muscle is trained to work more efficiently.

• Muscular endurance, or the ability of muscles to overcome the resistance for a prolonged period of time.

• Flexibility, to lengthen the muscles and increase the range of movement.

• Motor fitness, which includes such factors as agility, balance, reaction time, co-ordination, power and speed.

Running is rightly promoted as an ideal activity to increase cardio-vascular fitness. A balanced training programme, which includes regular stretching and work with weights, will also address the other four components of fitness which are less involved in the act of running itself. However, running when applying the principles of Alexander Technique – in other words, reading and absorbing

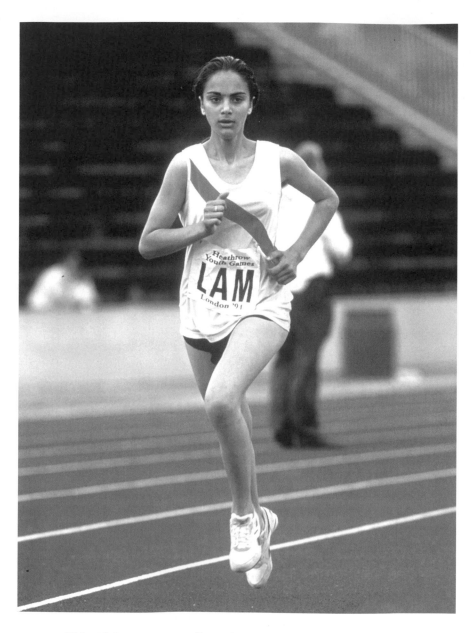

*This girl demonstrates excellent poise, awareness and economy of style,
showing how running can be transformed into an activity offering 'total fitness'.*

the information contained in this book! – transforms the sport into a means to acquire total fitness. This, say Cullum and Mowbray, 'is a far higher ideal than any of its parts. It is a state of being rather than doing, and available to all regardless of skill level, movement quality, body type, sex or any other hereditary or environmental influence. Possessing total fitness enables you to live rather than exist in our western culture. If total fitness is your aim, you will have to develop an independence of attitude that makes you self-reliant; you will exercise because you value fitness, not because you are told to exercise.'

CASE HISTORY – TOM

Tom took up running at the precocious age of 55 as a means of staying fit. Things went well for a few years, but then he started suffering from various injuries, particularly around his left hip. He began working with Paul Collins, an Alexander Technique teacher and ultra-marathoner who offered a course called 'The Art of Running'. Tom found that by applying some of the principles he learnt, such as 'practise the silent footfall', 'cultivate a beginner's mind' and 'lengthen up', his injury problems cleared and as a bonus he set several personal-bests.

Tom's story doesn't end there. Because he had found a way to run with more freedom and lightness, he reckoned he'd 'cracked it' and that he knew it all. Ten days before the London Marathon, he felt a little niggle in his left hip, but thought that if he rested it he'd be fine. However, on race day the niggle became a throbbing pain by the 10k mark and he literally had to crawl to the finish line. A few weeks later, he consulted an orthopaedic surgeon who told him that he had severe and irreversible arthritis in his left hip, that he'd never run again, and that he'd be back in 12 months for a hip replacement.

Tom decided to see if he could sort himself out, so twice a day he worked for an hour in front of a mirror, relearning how to walk according to the principles learnt from Paul Collins. He kept reminding himself, 'free the neck and lengthen up'. Within three months he was able to manage some light jogging and several months later completed a marathon! Two years after that, Tom wrote to tell me that he had just come third in his age category in the 80-mile South Downs Way Run, covering the distance in under 20 hours. Quite remarkable. Tom adds that without focusing all the time on the principle of 'lengthen up', he doesn't think he would even have finished the race, much less achieved third place.

WHY RUN?

We have already established that running is among the most efficient routes to cardio-vascular fitness. What are its other benefits?

• It's accessible. You can literally run anywhere, in towns or in the countryside, on a beach or up a mountain.

• It's cheap. Apart from a good pair of shoes, there's no other essential equipment.

• It's flexible. You can fit running around your lifestyle, and you don't need a partner or ten other team members to participate.

• It's a great way to keep weight under control. Few activities burn calories more quickly. For women, the areas of greatest weight loss are round the waist and hips.

• It's a superb stress-buster. A steady-paced run in a pleasant setting will soothe away the day's mental aches.

• It can reduce the risk of osteoporosis. Bones become porous and brittle with age, and calcium loss is proportionate to the level of (in)activity. Weight-bearing exercise such as running helps make them more dense and resilient. This is extremely important for women, who are more prone to osteoporosis than men due to the impact of the menopause.

• It's for all ages. There is no age at which it's too late to start running. The legendary Madge Sharples completed her first marathon in her 80s.

• It makes you feel good! Like all exercise, regular running induces a sense of well-being, and boosts self-esteem and confidence.

HOW OFTEN?

'Three times a week for at least 20 minutes' is the traditional prescription for the amount of exercise needed to generate fitness benefits. However, recent

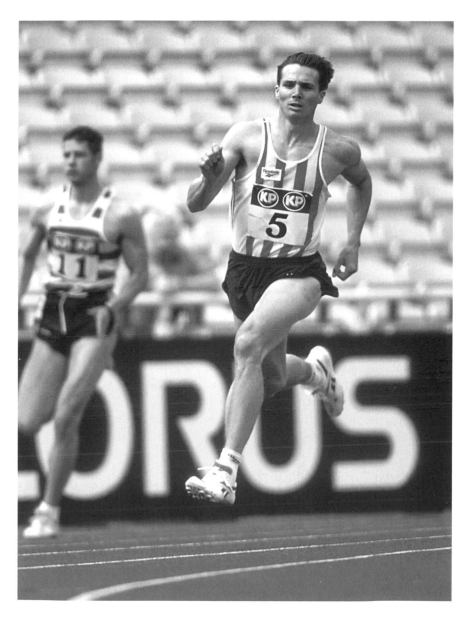

Roger Black offers the ideal combination in a competitive athlete:
power, control, focus and attention to form.

thinking has moved away from this rather dogmatic approach, with people now encouraged to build as much activity into their everyday lives as possible, be it walking to work, climbing stairs rather than using the lift, or digging the garden. This is fine as a way of coaxing couch potatoes into a more active lifestyle without them necessarily realising it, but runners may prefer the old formula – perhaps aiming for four outings per week of different duration and pace, preceded and followed by a ten-minute, low-intensity warm-up and cool-down with appropriate stretches.

TRAINING LEVELS

Whether you're running for fitness or competitively, it's important to know the intensity at which you're training. A simple way to monitor intensity is the 'talk test'. If you can maintain a conversation during your workout then you are not exceeding the ability of your aerobic system to provide your working muscles with the oxygen they require. When you start to gasp, then you are going too fast!

Another way to judge running intensity is to measure your heart rate. First, you need to work out your maximum heart rate (MHR). This can be measured precisely under laboratory conditions, although a good rough guide is to subtract your age from 220. Then keep a check on your heart rate to ensure that you are exercising at the appropriate level. The most accurate way is to buy a heart rate monitor that straps across the chest and gives readings on a digital watch worn on the wrist. Easier and cheaper is to feel the pulse in the carotid (neck) or radial (wrist) artery, using the index and middle finger (never the thumb). Count the beats for 15 seconds and multiply by four.

• 'Healthy heart zone' is 50-60 per cent of MHR, and is the level at which complete beginners, the seriously overweight or people in cardiac rehabilitation should be exercising. Brisk walking is an ideal fat-burner for this group.

• 'Fitness zone' is 60-70 per cent of MHR, producing a significant fat-burning effect due to its greater intensity. Gentle jogging will achieve this zone.

• 'Training zone' is 70-80 per cent of MHR, and is the level giving most general fitness benefits. Steady running with your heart rate in the training zone will improve your cardio-vascular and respiratory system (aerobic fitness) while increasing the size and strength of your heart. The higher intensity means more overall calories are burned, although fewer of these are from fat (low-intensity exercise is best for fat-burning).

- 'Anaerobic zone' is 80-90 per cent of MHR, and is the level to improve your V0₂ max (the highest amount of oxygen one can consume during exercise) and lactate tolerance (ability to fight the fatigue caused by the build-up of lactic acid). This is hard work, and only élite runners would want to work at this level for long periods.

- 'Red-line zone' is 90-100 per cent of MHR, and is as tough as it gets. Few can exercise at this level – the closest the rest of us might manage is during interval training, when steady work in the training zone is alternated with very short and controlled bursts of activity (no more than one minute) in the red-line zone.

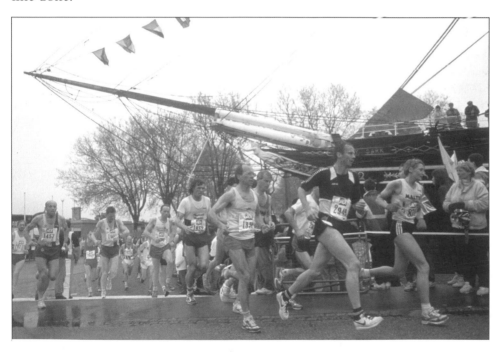

The London Marathon masses reach the Cutty Sark, less than a third of the way round the course: constant attention to form is vital if these athletes are to reach the finishing line.

4. FIT FOR ANYTHING?

It is now twenty years since Jane Fonda beseeched the world to 'go for the burn' and the global fitness phenomenon known as aerobics was born. As exercise advice, Fonda's famous dictum was soon shown to be suspect. However, the philosophy behind it was unimpeachable: *The Jane Fonda Workout Book* declared that we ordinary mortals were free to discover the physical, mental and social benefits of regular exercise – and that there was nothing wrong with trying to push ourselves that little bit harder. The age of legwarmers and lycra was upon us.

At the same time as Fonda and her followers were devising the basic routines of exercise to music and launching classes in church halls, dance studios and sports centres, there came a parallel boom in running. The oldest and most natural sport in the world had, for most of the 20th century, been the preserve of organised athletics clubs. But at the end of the 1970s, a dour decade of economic austerity and political upheaval on both sides of the Atlantic, the sport quickly gained popularity for similar reasons to aerobics: it was a cheap, accessible and flexible way to improve cardio-vascular fitness. Aerobics and running were available to both sexes and all ages, required no previous experience, and demanded little in the way of expensive memberships or specialist equipment.

Running transcended politics, class, creed and colour, so it was hardly surprising that the ultimate symbolic run – the 26 miles 385 yards of the marathon – became the holy grail for many participants. After taking part in the New York Marathon, Chris Brasher was inspired to create an equally democratic event in London. The race was founded in 1981 and, four years later, attracted a staggering 70,000 applications for 22,000 places. A decade later, more than 130 marathons were staged in the UK. But perhaps the most profound illustration of running's potential as a force for social cohesion came in May 1986, when almost one million people took part in six-mile runs throughout the UK, to raise money for famine relief in Africa through the charity Sport Aid.

POLITICS OF FATNESS

It was a popular notion during the late 1980s that the Western world was entering a new, liberated era, where greater quantities of free time and disposable income would enable more people to pursue their interests and, as a consequence, enjoy better health. However, it has turned out to be completely wrong. Despite constant massaging of the figures, the trend in unemployment has been generally upwards – thus disenfranchising a greater proportion of the population from the means to improve their health and well-being, such as a better diet and access to exercise. In addition, technological advances have meant that those in work are now compelled to put in ever longer hours, just to keep pace. The consequences for the health of a nation are obvious. Membership of fitness clubs has reached a plateau, while 80 per cent of people who make a New Year resolution to shape up are slumped back in their armchairs by March. A plethora of statistics offer damning evidence that Britain and America are becoming fat, idle societies keener to search for a miracle diet pill than to take regular, health-giving exercise.

In the United States, the National Institutes of Health (NIH) have promoted obesity from 'contributing risk factor' to 'major risk factor' for heart disease. 'Obesity has become a life-long disease, not a cosmetic issue, nor a moral judgement – and it is becoming a dangerous epidemic,' says Robert Eckel, an endocrinologist who heads the American Heart Association's nutrition committee. An alarming 55 per cent of the American population – 97 million people – are classed as 'overweight', of whom 38 million are 'obese' (which means a man standing 178 cm/5'10" weighing more than 94.6 kg/209 lbs). The total annual obesity bill in the US is $100 billion, including more than $51 billion in direct medical costs.

Meanwhile, obesity in Britain has doubled in the last 20 years, making its population the pudgiest in Europe. In 1999, according to the International Obesity Task Force, 17 per cent of men and 20 per cent of women were defined as clinically obese, which means having a body-mass index greater than 30. This is obtained by dividing your weight in kilograms by your height in metres, squared. A BMI of 20-25 is considered acceptable. There is now twice the incidence of obesity in Britain compared to France, Sweden and the Netherlands. 'We are in the lead of other European countries,' says Dr Andrew Hill, chairman of the Association for the Study of Obesity in Britain, 'but we are still about 15 years behind America'. Which is no reason to rest awhile, hands on our amply covered hips: further research has suggested that British teenagers are turned off sport because they think it is 'uncool', with girls particularly reluctant to partake in physical activity due to fears about their image. Despite major 'come and try it' projects mounted by organisations like the Sports Council (now Sport England) and the Health Education Authority, supported by well-known personalities as role models, it is clear that the next generation is no more likely to recognise the importance of taking regular exercise than the current one.

QUALITY TIME

Perhaps, then, it is the type of exercise which is the problem? The fitness boom of the mid- to late-1980s was accompanied by the creation of a very definite image, to suit the mood of the times: people who worked out were sleek, sophisticated, fashionable and attractive. However, these were all superficial attributes – little attention was paid to the inner motivations for exercise. Likewise, there was scant concern for the quality of the exercise performed. All that mattered was the number of repetitions, how much poundage, how many classes. With the benefit of hindsight and greater knowledge, it is now easy to question the value of an approach which had the capacity to be boring, repetitious and potentially hazardous – and also, in extreme cases, could lead to addiction, with obsessive Type 'A' personalities continuing to exercise when injured, refusing to take rest days and suffering withdrawal symptoms if deprived of their endorphin high.

Looking back, this was a mindlessly mechanical approach. It suddenly seemed rather pointless to spend 30 minutes pedalling on a bike with no wheels, or to pound the treadmill in a sweaty bunker when fresh air and sunshine were but a stride away. Magazines such as *Men's Health* were instrumental in reclaiming the great outdoors, and highlighting the tedium of a gym-based fitness programme. Walking, swimming and, indeed, running – activities deemed too staid for the thrusting 1980s executive – were back in fashion. As a result, those lacking the time or the money to join a swish fitness club were liberated from the tyranny of corporate membership.

This change of emphasis compelled the clubs to rethink their strategy. It was no longer acceptable to provide a weights room and an unvarying diet of high-impact aerobics classes and demand a four-figure sum for the privilege of access. Increasing professionalisation within the fitness industry, linked to higher expectations among customers, powered the second major revolution: a holistic approach to exercise.

HOLISTIC FITNESS

It is now difficult to find a major fitness centre on either side of the Atlantic that does not include the likes of yoga, tai chi and Pilates on its programme. Little more than a decade ago, these were esoteric pursuits, known only to a small band of initiates and undiscovered by the media. At the start of the new century, they have moved into the exercise mainstream, valued as techniques which embrace the idea of holism.

The term 'holistic' comes from the Greek word for 'whole', and was coined in the 1920s to describe any system, be it medicine or exercise, that considers the whole person – body, mind and spirit – within the wider environment of family, culture and community. The basic principles are that each individual is unique; that the psycho-social aspects of lifestyle and personal fulfilment are essential to good health; and that practitioner and client share responsibility for the success of the process. In *Holistic Health: How to Understand and Use the Revolution in Medicine*, Lawrence LeShan offered an analogy comparing the methods of the gardener and the mechanic: 'The gardener deals with the whole – with the organism in an environment. The mechanic fixes non-functioning parts'. This analogy can be extended further: the gym supervisor offers instruction in how to build big biceps. The Alexander teacher, in contrast, works with the client on a mutual journey of psycho-physical self-discovery.

In his excellent book *The Owner's Guide to the Body*, Roger Golten prefers the term 'somatic' to 'holistic' – the word, appropriately, is Greek for 'body'. He includes Alexander Technique in a list of activities, along with yoga, tai chi and others, as examples of somatic education which form what he calls 'the new gym'. The main characteristic of somatic education is the active participation of the client in the process, with the therapist/coach acting as guide and facilitator. 'In this model,' Golten writes, 'hard is no longer good, and harder better, although tone and strength are valued. The new gym works from the inside out: the emphasis is on releasing tension, stretching short or tight tissues, relating the mind and body, self-understanding, self-care, self-acceptance, self-expression, posture and the quality rather than the quantity of what you've got.

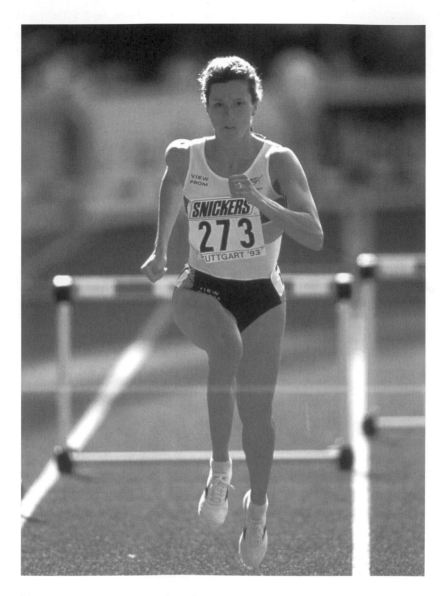

*Now retired from the track and involved in health promotion initiatives, the challenge
facing former 400 metres hurdles world champion and Olympic gold medallist
Sally Gunnell is to encourage girls to recognise the importance of taking regular exercise.*

Somatic education is about connecting us to ourselves, mind to body and body-mind to spirit.' By embracing the demand for types of exercise which require thought, analysis and interaction, the fitness industry has undergone the most satisfying revolution of all.

ALEXANDER TECHNIQUE AND SWIMMING

Perhaps the most fascinating link between a conventional fitness activity and a holistic/somatic approach has been in swimming, exemplified by Steven Shaw and Armand D'Angour's book *The Art of Swimming*.

A competitive swimmer in his youth, Shaw quit the sport at 17 bored and exhausted. When he started learning Alexander Technique, his teacher suggested that the years of swimming were the main cause of residual stiffness in his upper torso. Shaw returned to the pool to find out. He became aware of the damaging efforts he exerted in pulling his head back in his favoured breast stroke. 'I also noted,' he writes in the book, 'that my competitive instincts were so ingrained that I couldn't let myself be overtaken, but would strain to stay ahead of other swimmers at all costs! Learning to check these habits and "slow down" presented the challenge of discovering a new kind of self-control. It opened up for me an exciting new dimension, a sense of continuing exploration of the water and of myself.'

The question posed by Shaw and D'Angour's book is whether swimming can be an art. They argue convincingly that it can, by downplaying the need to swim faster or further in favour of swimming well and enjoying the water. Instead of making efficient swimming sound like rocket science, and turning competitive swimming into 'a battle against an intransigent opponent', the process of exploration and the 'pleasure of enhanced awareness in the water' should be the rewards of the activity.

The process by which traditional sports and contemporary theories of exercise draw together is certain to continue, since much of sport has remained hermetically sealed for decades, suspicious and fearful of innovation. Perhaps the barriers are finally coming down?

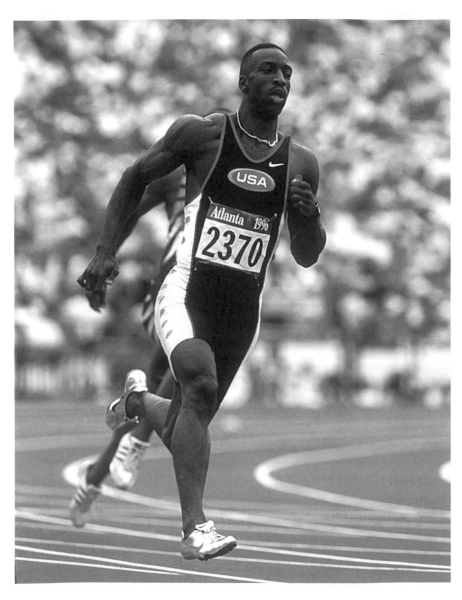

*Michael Johnson demonstrating his unique way of 'running tall',
proving that freedom is a condition not a position.*

5. HOW TO RUN WELL

The mind, drilled and grilled to wrong concepts, reacts against itself. The result is that as the athlete tries hard, the power exerted is transferred to his antagonistic muscles. The harder he tries, the more his brakes pull on.

Percy Cerutty

When we see a great runner, or a youngster (more often a girl than a boy because boys tend to copy their idols and lose some of their fluency), flowing along in full stride, we witness a connection with the sublime. But how can we capture what sports psychologists refer to as 'peak experience' or 'being in the zone'?

Alexander believed that we can no longer rely on our instincts to guide us correctly or accurately in our activities. Part of the reason for this is that many people do not have a clear or correct idea of how to do things, of what is required and, more importantly, what isn't.

Take, for example, the way most people sit down. They begin by shortening the neck and pulling the head back, which compresses the spine. Then they aim their bum towards the chair, causing the lower back to stiffen and arch. Then they drop their weight – in other words, collapse – into the chair.

Common responses as to why they sit in this way range from: 'I'm afraid the chair won't be there' to 'I'm trying to keep my balance'. In fact, most people have forgotten (if they ever really knew) what is needed to sit. Instead, they rely on a conception that is built from their experience. Anyone who has ever done any Alexander Technique work knows that this old conception can be replaced with something that is much more free and unconstricted, and which respects the way we are actually designed.

So how *are* we designed to bend? Watch a two-year-old pick up his/her toys to see an example of natural, undistorted movement. In the course of Alexander Technique lessons, the pupil learns a new concept of bending along the lines of the head, leading the spine into length, while the knees release out over the toes and the pupil then finds him/herself sitting in the chair. Faulty or inaccurate beliefs about how one gets from A to B affect runners, too:

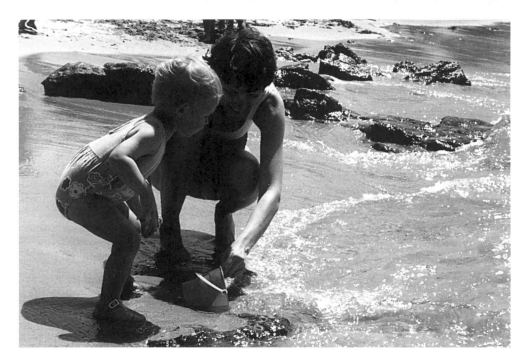

Most small children provide good examples of free and undistorted movement.

• **Running is done with the legs.** At first, this statement would seem so obvious as to border on the ridiculous, as in, 'Of course we run with the legs. If we didn't have legs we couldn't run'. Consider, then, the view of Percy Cerutty, the late Australian Olympic coach, who said: 'You run on the legs not with them'.

Runners who run *with* their legs tend to do more than is necessary in order to move. Rather than flowing, they do a lot of pushing and shoving, and their leg action lacks the fluidity and smoothness we see in great athletes or ten-year-old girls. They may push themselves upwards rather than rolling forwards, under the mistaken belief that running fast requires this kind of effort. They tend to focus on contracting their legs rather than releasing them, specifically the front of the ankles and the back of the knees, thereby forcing muscles to work against each other. They may pound, or run *into* the ground rather than *over* it, thereby contributing to the lower-leg problems that plague runners at all levels.

- **The legs and particularly the feet should lead the movement.** If a runner believes this (and it's a not-uncommon idea, by the way), this tends to make the runner work against him/herself and fight against gravity rather than using it for his/her benefit. The runner will lean back and tighten in order not to fall, with the feet extending in front and pulling him/her along.

In contrast to these faulty and inaccurate beliefs, here are some of the key components in learning how to run well:

- **Good runners run tall.** They don't hunch or lean.

- **They run with the brakes off.** There is an economy and an integrity in their form and movement.

- **They run smoothly.** While the smoothest runner does not always get to the line first, s/he still represents the ideal to which we can aspire. I may not have looked like Joachim Cruz in full flight but, as my own use improved, my form did likewise: longer stride, longer spine, head not retracted, better use of the arms.

- **Less can equal more.** Coaches in a variety of sports are now emphasising the importance of quality rather than quantity as the key to improvement and greater all-round fitness. The same theme, incidentally, is echoed by many musicians.

- **If you listen to the whispers you won't have to hear the screams.** Runners, like musicians, often train through and into injuries. On many occasions, a small niggle, if paid attention to, disappears. This enables a runner to survive and even thrive on the stresses imposed by high-quality training. However, as the saying goes, 'Those who don't learn will be taught' – and the lesson could be very painful. Running when injured or ill, for example, may have disastrous consequences.

• **Runners who pound often end up injured.** Good runners run lightly, they don't try and excavate holes in the ground with each stride.

• **Have confidence in the process and enjoy it more.** Alexander's belief that by paying attention to the means, the ends will take care of themselves, allowed me to take each day as it came when applied to the regimes of training and racing. I began to understand that I didn't need to put in extra workouts – and as for the tougher sessions, which can produce a lot of anxiety, I started to see them as opportunities to learn. How do I react to the worry of striving for a target time, or cope with the pain which this might cause? How can I enjoy the camaraderie of my fellow runners, and take satisfaction from completing something that seemed impossible half-an-hour earlier?

MY STORY – TOM

At the age of 18, I was ranked fifth fastest in the world over 1,500 metres as an under-20. I was faster than the world number two Noah Ngeny. I was also British junior cross-country champion, and went on to represent Great Britain in both the world track and cross-country championships. I had been a junior international for four years prior to this.

My first opportunity to race at world level came two years after my junior successes (and also after six stress fractures), at a grand prix meeting in Rieti. Facing the world mile record-holder Noureddine Morceli, I led the pace through 500 metres – a sharp lesson learnt, as I then faded! Since then I have watched and raced against many world-class athletes, and also seen some of the training they do. It is amazing to see how much time they spend correcting their running style. I know Wilson Kipketer (800 metres world record-holder) and the Moroccans, especially Salah Hissou (former 10 kilometres world record-holder), will devote hours to improving their technique.

That year, I went on to run 3 min 41.2 secs for 1,500 metres and in my first-ever mile ran 4 min 00.02 secs! Injury has dogged my career, but I was eventually rewarded with a senior international vest to run the 1,500 metres against France. I am still Britain's number one under-23, and fifth fastest as a senior. I am only young, 6'3" and 76 kg, and I have experience and good performances behind me – all I need now is to sustain a year of training without injury to get back to where I should be. That is the reason for becoming a full-time athlete.

This is a typical training week:

> Monday am: 5 miles, easy.
> Monday pm: 5 miles, easy.
> Tuesday am: 5 miles, steady.
> Tuesday pm: Interval work: 10 x 400 metres with one minute recovery in-between, aiming for 60 seconds or under.
> Wednesday am: 9-10 miles, easy.
> Wednesday pm: Strength training.
> Thursday am: 5 miles, easy.
> Thursday pm: Hill work.
> Friday: Rest or two easy runs.
> Saturday am: Interval work: 1,000m, 800m, 600m, 400m, 200m (with three minutes recovery in-between).
> Saturday pm: 5 miles, easy.
> Sunday am: 10-15 miles, easy.
> Sunday pm: Strength training/plyometrics.

My schedule is based mainly on years of trial and error, and also scientific input from my coach (dad). I have built up to this over the past four months and it is going well. I have never worked at this intensity before, as my shins used to ache and then fracture. Now, though, they don't – maybe I have finished growing and have the proper physical structure.

It has been almost four years since I started Alexander Technique lessons. Initially I was more concerned with the potential benefits that Alexander Technique would have on my performance and running style, thinking that it would directly influence my times and personal bests. In short, it did – I have not been running so well for years.

However, it was the effects of Alexander Technique on racing and training that enabled me to go faster. I now train more efficiently, so ultimately I can do more. If I don't want to do more, then I can do the same work but with less effort. I call it 'efficiency and economy of motion'. In short, I can recover more quickly. This means that I can train without strain: be as relaxed on the last repetition in interval sessions as on the first, be fresh each time I run, push myself further than before without breaking down, and recover sufficiently when I run twice or even three times a day. If I go beyond the boundaries of efficient training, my body starts to tell me through fatigue and injury.

This process is vital feedback. It has taken me a long time to learn which feed-back to heed, but I never stop listening to my body now as it tells me every-thing: am I hungry? Am I tired? Am I ill? So I listen. All this stems from the simple Alexander Technique directions, and shedding the bad habits and pat-terns that got in the way of the feedback.

I now feel so fresh and recover so quickly that I get back home wanting to go training again. I enjoy the freedom, I cruise without effort, sometimes I even float. To me, that is training. The body moves, and I simply tell it which direction.

HOW TO RUN BADLY

A simple definition of fanaticism is 'redoubling your efforts when you've lost sight of your goal'. We all accept that in order to improve, you need to try hard. But this belief is often very effective at feeding the 'end-gaining' monster that is lurking, ready to take over your life. Here are a few signs that it may have done so:

● You work to the principle that 'more is more'. More mileage, more effort, more speed, more vitamins, more shoes…

● You ignore the warning signs and believe that 'no pain, no gain' is an ideal philosophy for training, as well as for life.

● You always run hard and compete whenever possible, especially in training. You try never to let anyone finish in front of you, even on 'easy' days.

● You become obsessed with having to run so many miles or for so many min-utes each day and insist on telling anyone and everyone about it.

● As a 43-year-old male (replace age, sex, distance and goal to suit your own circumstances), your entire life and sense of well-being hinge on your break-ing 47 mins for 10k.

● You train every day, never take a day off, and view walking, stopping to enjoy the view or to smell the flowers as a sign of weakness.

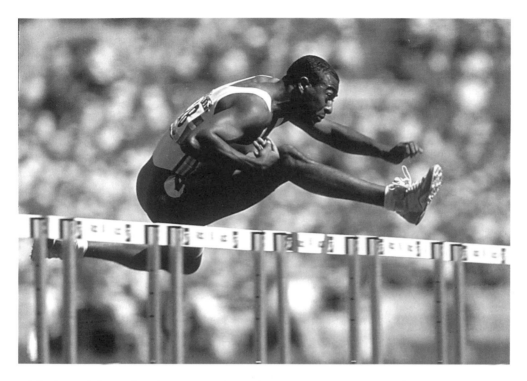

The do's and don'ts of good running apply equally to those athletes competing in more technical events, as shown by Colin Jackson during the 110 metres hurdles at the 1988 Seoul Olympic Games.

RUNNING DO'S AND DON'TS: A SUMMARY

—Do's

• **Allow the arms to engage the legs.** The shoulders need to remain free so that the movement of the arms can connect with the legs through the back.

• **Allow the ankles to release, followed by a release towards the back of the knees.** In order to allow the knees to bend freely — that is, without having to overcome any self-induced resistance — the ankles need to be free. Ask a friend to hold on to your ankle and try to bend your knee. You will need to work hard to overcome the resistance. When they let go, the knee bends more easily. Any holding in the ankles will make a smooth stride less likely.

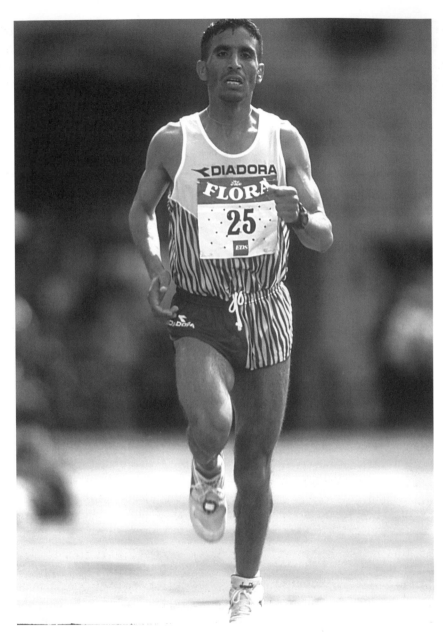

'Let the eyes look out 30-50 metres ahead':
Abdelkhader El Mouaziz during the 1998 Flora London Marathon.

• **Allow the knees rather than the feet to lead the movement forward.** Trying to increase stride length by reaching forward with the foot results in a braking action which will slow you down. It also causes a runner to lean back or sit on their hips rather than run tall. Instead, let the knee lead the leg forward and stride length will come as a result of the foot extending behind you.

• **Allow the legs to move in a semi-circular pattern.** Good runners allow their legs to turn over in a semi-circular fashion, with the heel approaching the buttock at the end of each stride (that is, the knee bends at least 90° before coming forward). Thinking of the legs moving in a circular rather than a linear way helps a runner to develop a rhythmic pattern which is easier to maintain and to modify according to need, such as increasing speed or running uphill.

• **Remember that the external direction is forward, the internal direction is up.** Many runners need to understand that although they may be moving forward in space, their spine does not have to aim the same way. Ideally, as you are moving forward (that is, horizontally), as a result of the action of your legs and feet, your spine should be lengthening upwards (that is, vertically), with the head leading the way. This upward tendency produces a lightness in the body, which means the legs do not have to work so hard to move you forward – and, as my mother used to say, 'You get more bang for your buck'. When a runner's spine goes forward instead of up, by pushing the chest or pelvis towards the target, a downward shortening tendency in the back is encouraged, as well as a quality of heaviness – all of which is compensated by the legs working much harder than they need to.

• **Let the eyes look out 30–50 metres ahead.** Not only will you see more of the countryside, cityscape or parkland, but running with a lengthened spine and a poised head will encourage balance and reduce both 'heavy' running and much of the strain on neck and shoulders.

Warning: looking out if the eyes are fixed will require the runner to tighten the neck and pull the head back in order to get the eyes into the right plane – not good. Our gaze can be shifted independently of head movement. Allow your eyes to move as your head remains lightly poised atop your spine.

• **Allow the wrists to remain toned rather than floppy.** Runners mistakenly run with their wrists so loose that their hands flop around, in the belief that they are relaxed in so doing. They are, in fact, creating unnecessary tension elsewhere as the shoulders will often tighten to pick up the slack. Instead, runners should allow enough tone in their wrists to maintain them in a stable relationship between the hand and arm. Stiff thumbs are another indication that there is too much tension.

● **Allow the elbows to remain bent at 90 degrees.** This is a very efficient way to organise the arms. While variations on this set-up are not a sin, remember that a short lever is more efficient as it requires less energy to move. Since we want the arms to participate and contribute to the running action, we need to know how this can be done as effectively and smoothly as possible.

● **Allow the arms to move straight forward and back or slightly across the body.** Runners do a lot of interesting things with their arms. Some movements contribute more to propelling you forward than others: the most effective is when the arms move forward and back more or less in a straight line. When we say 'arm', we really mean the forearm. A sprinter's forearm will be parallel to the ground both when it swings forward and when it is pulled back. Runners moving less quickly should modify the range of motion to match their speed and terrain (less on the flat, more going uphill).

Another point to note: the effort comes in bringing the arm back, not in pushing it forward. Bringing the arm back helps the legs pull you forward (via the back).

● **Learn to run lightly and quietly.** Pounding (some refer to this as digging holes or excavating) is a sign that something's wrong. You may be tired, not feeling well or simply not paying attention. Running lightly has nothing to do with how much you weigh, as anyone with children who like to run around when you are trying to take a nap will attest. It has much more to do with attention (listening to yourself as you run) and intention (thinking 'up').

When runners pound, they literally jar their whole system and can be blamed for much of the bad press the activity has received in recent years. For example, running has been accused of causing the uterus to drop and being bad for the spine, and various low-impact alternatives are often recommended. The Alexandrian saying, 'It's not what you do, it's the way that you do it', has some relevance here. The question we need to ask is: which qualities support our capacity to make running a pleasure, and which do the opposite?

• **Run on the legs, not with the legs.** I think Percy Cerutty meant that when runners over-emphasise the legs, an imbalance is created and overall co-ordination is compromised. In Alexander terms, the primary pattern is the head-neck-back and the legs are a secondary pattern. This means that the movement of the legs should not cause undue disbuggerance, as Patrick Macdonald used to say, to the head-neck-back relationship.

The Italian concept appaggio, normally used in the context of voice training, sheds some light on Cerutty's comment. Appaggio refers to our capacity to co-ordinate ourselves in such an efficient way that the function of any of our muscles is not violated by the exaggerated action of another. In other words, efficient running depends on our ability to co-ordinate the action of the legs with the movement of the arms and torso (see *Let's Twist Again* in Chapter 6 for more about this relationship). Cerutty was no doubt aware (as any Alexandrian knows) that lack of movement in the torso does not mean a lack of activity.

MY STORY – GUY

I used to do a lot of jogging years ago and really enjoyed it, even though I was dissatisfied with my style and felt I was too heavy to be a decent runner. It was a good way of getting outside and setting my body in motion, which always brought me great relief.

Eventually, though, I decided to stop because I realised it was hurting my back. I didn't blame my poor technique, I simply thought that jogging was bad for me – that I was destroying my spine for the sake of keeping in shape, and that it made no sense. At the time, I had no idea that it was possible to 'learn to run'. So I gave up jogging altogether and developed an interest in alternative therapies and body awareness techniques, with the goal of reducing muscular tension and generally lowering my anxiety level.

During that quest, I read about the Alexander Technique but never felt attracted to it until a couple of years ago, when it became clear to me that I had to change the position of my head relative to the rest of my body. At my first lesson, which was a group session with Simon Ghiberti, I walked around the room while Simon lightly held my head to prevent me pulling it back and down. Suddenly, I began to breathe beautifully – a sensation so delicious that I definitely wanted to learn more. I took weekly lessons with Simon for about a year and was making steady progress, but I wanted to apply the Technique in a more active way, possibly to training activities.

I had seen the picture of Michael Gelb holding the neck of a student while running next to him, and I wanted to try something like that. So when I learned that Malcolm Balk was an Alexander Technique teacher, a competitive runner and also a coach, I decided it was time for a change. At first, we worked mostly on walking, sitting, standing and other daily activities. I was astonished by his ability to read my body's history. He knew at once that I was doing body-building. Later on, he asked me if I had done a lot of swimming, which was actually true. After a few months, we went outside for the first time to work on running and I gradually re-introduced jogging to my life.

A year has passed since then, and I have to say that I am pleased with the results. First of all, I no longer have to worry about hurting my back: because I make better use of my body, the impact of the steps on my spine is greatly reduced, and I don't have the feeling of being 'crooked' that I used to have after a run. Next, I feel a lot lighter while I am running: my steps are quicker and my feet seem to brush against the ground instead of pounding on it like they used to. This is a nice contrast to my previous feelings of heaviness and clumsiness, which I thought was part of my quintessential nature.

The last aspect is a simple extension of the first two: if I can learn to run with lightness, could I not also learn to live that way? How can this knowledge that I have acquired about running be applied to the rest of my life? Now, isn't that an interesting project?

—Don'ts

• **Push the body up and let it land heavily on the legs with every stride.** Pushing the body upwards takes a great deal of effort which may be useful in a training context (to strengthen the legs, for example) but is an inefficient way to move a runner forward. Some runners mistakenly believe that pushing themselves up with the legs helps them run taller. In fact, it tends to a) stiffen the legs; b) do little to increase overall height, which is a function of the length of the spine; and c) waste valuable time and energy.

• **Push with the feet.** A lot of runners think that it is necessary to push with the feet in order to run. This habit is unnecessary because there is plenty of friction between foot and ground (especially with today's high-tech shoes) to move the runner forward without the need for extra effort. Adding the push often interferes with co-ordination and puts strain on the foot/ankle/calf, which can lead to pain or injury. Some coaches recommend a toe flick at the end of the push-off phase (just before the flight phase when both feet are off the ground) as a way of increasing power and stride length. This is fine as long as it is timed properly, helps move the runner forward (rather than up), and doesn't lead to a stiffening of the legs.

• **Lock the arms on to the trunk or fix the shoulders.** We often see runners who have allowed their arms to become heavy and unenergised, so that they do not move as easily or freely as they should. The arms then function as weights, which serve to pull the runner down into a moving slouch. The problem does not necessarily originate with the arms, but can be traced back to a poor head-neck relationship. Thinking about freeing (not holding) the armpits can help release the arms and allow them to move more easily. This direction also helps to reduce tension and pain in the shoulder blade/lower neck area, which some runners suffer from time to time.

• **Allow the feet to cross over the mid-line.** Some runners like to let their feet cross over the imaginary line running between them, a habit which leads to the upper body swaying back and forth. This also throws the hips from side to side, as anyone who has seen or mimicked the model's catwalk stride will know. The runner must then use extra effort and energy to adjust to all this rock-and-roll.

• **Do an Elvis, and tuck or push the pelvis into the legs.** Runners, especially those who arch their lower backs, are often advised to do what is referred to in some circles as the 'pelvic tuck', where the buttocks are tightened and the pelvis is tucked under. The intention of this advice is to help reduce the excessive curve in the lower back. Unfortunately, this measure often causes unwanted side-effects: for example, tucking the pelvis can produce a downward pull which must be countered with muscular effort elsewhere, often in the form of pulling up the sternum. This tightens and narrows the lower back, fixes the ribs and makes it hard to breathe and to move the legs. In effect, a type of internal civil war is created, with one part of the body at odds with another: the pelvis trying to pull the back down and the sternum striving desperately to resist.

Another side-effect is for runners to push the pelvis into the legs when they run. What does this mean? Try a little experiment. Stand with your back touching a wall, feet about 5 cm from it. Your shoulders and bum should be in contact. Now bend your knees so that you slide down the wall about 30 cm. Is your bum still touching the wall, or has it come away, following the knees?

The same experiment can be done away from the wall with a friend standing beside you. Bend your knees and have your friend notice whether or not your back stays vertical or if you tend to lean backwards and push your pelvis forward. We are, in fact, designed to bend at the hip joint – which is not, contrary to popular belief, found in the waist but in the buttock, much lower. This means that the legs should move independently from the back, which includes the pelvis. In terms of direction, I like to think of the knees going forward and away while the back, including the pelvis, is encouraged to go back and up.

• **Allow the head to roll, bob, wag or look down.** Once you are aware that the head weighs about 4.5 kg (10 lbs), it doesn't take a rocket scientist to figure out that letting the head roll around is going to place a tremendous load on the rest of the body, beginning with the spine. Runners who allow their head to waggle are often under the false impression that this is a way to relax the neck. In contrast, it puts more strain on the neck, which must now work much harder to cope with the constant shifts in the balance of the head.

• **Allow the fists to clench, the wrists to flop and the thumbs to stiffen.** Too much tension or not enough tone in the hands and wrists contributes to similar problems elsewhere. Try, for example, to make a tight fist without tensing up the shoulders.

• **Clench the teeth or grimace.** Like musicians, runners do some pretty awful things with their jaws, teeth and faces when they run, especially when under stress. Besides the possibility of frightening small children, facial grimaces do little to help you get from A to B. In fact, they can be an indication that your energy is being misdirected rather than going where it will do most good.

• **Bounce up and down or roll from side to side.** Research has shown that élite runners have less vertical change in their centres of mass compared to average runners, and that reducing one's quantity of vertical movement tends to improve running economy. In other words, don't bounce up and down if you want to run with less effort.

● **Push the chest toward the target.** Alexander's dictum that 'the head leads and the body follows' is relevant here. When runners push their chest toward the target, the head tends to be thrown backwards, *away* from the target! Pushing or lifting the chest also tightens and hollows the back, which makes it harder to breathe naturally and leads to the following suggestion: belly breathing.

● **Belly-breathe.** It has been advocated in some circles that belly breathing is the correct way to breathe when running. Nothing could be further from the truth. However, it is safe to say that if a runner tries to run tall by lifting the chest, tucking the pelvis and thereby fixing the ribs, he or she may not have any choice! Try this experiment. Hold your lower ribs firmly with your hands and try to take a deep breath. You'll find that it's not easy. Now try slumping and taking a deep breath. The same, yes? In these circumstances, the runner's only option to gain a full breath is to over-expand the abdomen.

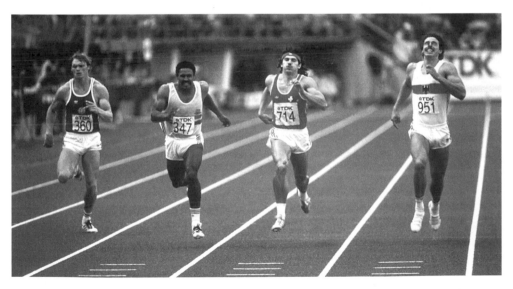

A fascinating study of disintegrating form! Such lapses in technique are, however, entirely understandable at the conclusion of the 400 metres, one of the most gruelling events in the decathlon.

6. APPLYING ALEXANDER

Alexander discovered that the way we 'use' ourselves affects the way we function. He was particularly interested in the role that the head-neck-back relationship, sometimes referred to as primary control, plays in this context. Alexander said that when the tone in the neck allows the head to be poised on top of the spine in such a way that the spine is encouraged to lengthen, then we function better and move more freely. We can observe the effects of a well-organised primary control in young children, great athletes (Muhammad Ali, Carl Lewis) and performers (Fred Astaire, Margot Fonteyn), and in many tribesmen and women.

Procedures used in Alexander Technique classes have several purposes. Chief of these is to focus attention on a specific pattern of movement within the context of general co-ordination. Alexander used arrangements he called 'positions of mechanical advantage' to encourage a general release, freedom and balance. For example, an attitude of standing with the body inclined a little forward, with hip, knee and ankle joints flexed, helps to encourage lengthening when bending – as opposed to the common tendency to compress and collapse in this activity.

The purpose is to promote 'good use' – that is, to reduce or eliminate extraneous movement, misdirected effort and unnecessary tension. This can only be good as far as runners are concerned! Here are some classic procedures (note that they should not be mistaken for exercises) plus a few of my own devising which runners, with or without the help of an Alexander Technique teacher, can practise now and again.

SEMI-SUPINE OR ACTIVE REST POSITION

The 'semi-supine' position, as it is now often termed (Alexander called it simply 'lying down'), is one of the most popular procedures taught in the

Alexander Technique – and deservedly so. In semi-supine the runner lies on a firm surface (a mattress or a sofa are too soft) in a warm and dry room (this may pose a challenge for some readers in the UK). Legs are bent with the knees pointing toward the ceiling while the hands rest on the lower abdomen with the elbows pointing out to the side. The back of the head is supported with a few books and the eyes should be left open. Lying in this position for ten minutes or so offers many benefits to the runner.

TEN GREAT REASONS FOR LYING DOWN

- **To let go of the day and release unnecessary tension.** Always useful!

- **To reconnect with one's body.** Awareness can be a wonderful thing for a runner. Except for the daily demands of stomach, bladder and lower intestine (and perhaps the odd nagging injury), runners may remain blissfully unaware of themselves. During lying-down work, a runner can wake up to what is happening with his/her body, giving an increased ability to respond effectively to feedback from within (sensations) and without (coach's instructions).

- **To increase balance and co-ordination.** While some might argue that runners are a bit unbalanced anyway, the fact remains that most could improve in this area. Try this simple test: stand in front of a mirror with your feet fairly close together. Now lift one knee so that you are standing, stork-like, on one leg. How much have you leaned over to one side? More than a degree or two indicates a problem as this gesture does not require any major adjustment. There should be no perceptible shift of weight to the supporting leg.

Balance sorts itself out, if we allow it to. We all possess a set of reflexes which will do the job providing we do not interfere with them!

One of the most common methods of 'getting in the way' has to do with how we carry our heads. If we allow the head to remain poised and free on top of the spine, then balance is greatly facilitated. Pull the head down, and we have to work much harder to achieve the same result. Hence the usefulness of lying-down work. Done properly, it can help to reduce the way we inadvertently interfere with the poise of the head – thereby eliminating one more obstacle from our path to greatness, a new personal-best or, at the very least, a more pleasant run.

- **To improve breathing.** For many runners (and other mortals), sitting usually involves a degree of collapse. In this state, the ribs which house the lungs end up practically on top of the pelvis, greatly reducing the capacity of the lungs to expand. Breathing then, as a matter of necessity, gets stuck up in the chest.

Slump in your seat and try to take a deep breath. Now sit up and repeat the process. For most people, breathing deeply is far easier in the second instance. While most runners do tend to reduce their normal 'slump' when they run, their breathing may still be laboured – and it's not because of the pace. Instead, the muscles which pull the ribs down have not fully released and have to be worked against. It's a bit like running in a t-shirt that's a couple of sizes too small. Lying down and getting the torso to release into lengthening and widening helps to remove this kind of restriction.

- **To give more length.** While running coaches the world over exhort their charges (with good reason) to 'run tall', the sad fact is that most tend to shorten themselves. Studies have shown that the average person tends to lose several centimetres in height between waking up in the morning and going to sleep at night. This is caused by pressure on the spinal discs, plus a tendency to pull down or collapse, which literally squeezes the juice out of our spines. This phenomenon can be lessened if we lie down and learn to lengthen ourselves, especially if done before noon (for you good runners who get up around 8am and go to bed well before midnight).

- **To enhance arousal, focus and attention levels.** Running well, particularly in competition, is related to what sports psychologists call 'arousal' (or if that sounds too sexy, 'activation level'). Too low and you feel sluggish, tired and unmotivated. Too high and you feel stressed, pressured and tense. Most athletes know when they are 'in the zone': energised, focused, ready and eager to run well. Lying down can help a runner become aware of how s/he is reacting to the upcoming event (for example, shallow breathing, tension in the neck and shoulders, worry about performing well) while creating the conditions for ideal performance (long spine, relaxed breathing, sense of control).

- **To achieve the transition from rest to activity**. Lying-down work can help smooth the transition from a sedentary to a more active state. Rather than forcing the body to respond to our wishes, we can help it prepare gently and thus reduce the chance of injury.

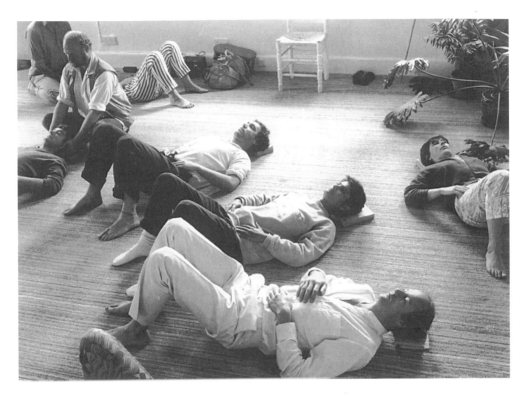

'Semi-supine' is one of the most popular procedures taught in the Alexander Technique, with particular benefits for runners.

● **To aid recovery.** Runners are not always aware of how they have tightened, pulled themselves down (shortened) or distorted their structure. Lying down after a workout will help an athlete to release the unnecessary tension and unwanted postural distortion built up during training. Left unchecked, these reactions can easily become part of the athlete's pattern of use and thus affect other areas of life.

● **To boost energy.** Most competitive runners are not full-time athletes, and can't afford to lounge around between workouts watching videos or playing computer games! They have to work, go to college, bring up a family, and so on. As a result, their energy may be depleted when it comes to training. A non-caffeinated method of rejuvenation is to lie down in a semi-supine position for around ten minutes.

• **To reawaken the lost sixth sense.** After taste, touch, smell, sight and hearing is the sixth sense of kinaesthesia – that which helps us to distinguish our arse from our elbow. Tense, over-contracted muscles, fixed joints and long periods of inactivity all tend to reduce this sixth sense, and with it our capacity to 'hear the whispers before they turn into screams'. According to David Garlick, 'As a person becomes aware of his/her muscle state, this lays the basis for better functioning of the musculo-skeletal system and will help to prevent or lessen musculo-skeletal problems. Secondly, there is an important effect psychologically in being aware, even if only every now and again, of one's muscles. There develops a sense of individual unity, of being at peace with oneself, of being "centered" in oneself.' Learning to release strongly contracted muscles through lying-down work helps undo our tendency to suppress sensory inputs and eases us back in touch with ourselves.

MY STORY – LARRY

When I began running in 1976, I had been cycling for several years and was in fairly good condition. I ran about two miles on my first outing and within three weeks had increased that to six miles. Although I had begun primarily to accompany a girlfriend, I soon fell in love with the simplicity and elegance of running and it became a regular part of my life.

Three years later, I was nearly finished with a four-mile run at steady tempo when I felt a cramp at the outside of my right knee. I tried to run through it, but the pain increased and I had to stop. After stretching for a few minutes, I was able to jog home. The knee felt fine at the beginning of my next run, but quickly tightened up after less than a mile. To make matters worse, the left knee had begun to cramp in the same manner.

I was soon unable to run at all, and decided to take some time off. Thus began a period of 12 years during which I was physically incapable of running. I tried everything: stretching, massage, acupuncture. I visited podiatrists, chiropractors, physiotherapists, but all to no avail. I resigned myself to my fate and continued cycling and swimming, but periodically would try to go for a run. Even if I had not done so for a full year, the cramping would recur within half a mile.

During this time I was pursuing a career in theatre and dance, performing highly demanding physical works and touring extensively abroad. I had taken some group Alexander Technique classes, but even though they were taught by a teacher trained by Alexander himself, they were not very profound and certainly did not help me to address my knee problem.

It was only when I saw the changes wrought in some friends by private lessons in the Technique that I became interested enough to do some reading and, eventually, to begin regular lessons. The changes came very quickly. After a matter of weeks, I decided to enrol to become a teacher of the Alexander Technique. I had been over-toned muscularly, but as this changed I was able to resolve many persistent problems including insomnia and tendon and joint inflammation.

Some time in my third year of training, I decided that I ought to be able to work out my running difficulties. I bought a new pair of shoes (yet again) and set out on a nice dirt road, primary control in mind. I soon began to feel the familiar twinges at my outer knees – but this time, what I was doing to cause the problem was as clear as day. I was lifting my foot as my leg recovered by contracting a long band of tendon and muscle (*peroneus longus*) that extends from the outer knee and wraps under the foot from its outer edge. I was therefore able to stop running, work on myself briefly and then continue, using primary control to alter the pattern. After about an hour of running, walking and stopping, I was able to prevent the misuse. After another two weeks I could run three miles, only occasionally stopping when I lost awareness of myself.

In retrospect, it was fortunate that I did not run during the time that I began my Alexander Technique studies. By the time I began to run again, I had changed sufficiently in the way that I used myself that the habitual misuse which was triggered by running was obvious to me – and, here is the good part, I was able to do something about it. Only with great discomfort could I allow myself to run as I had done in the past.

Remember, Alexander worked on sending directions for the optimal functioning of primary control for many months before he was able to sustain them while he attempted to speak. Let me go back, and give a more detailed description of the process that I went through in gaining control over my running difficulty.

In my Alexander Technique lessons, I had spent hours simply finding out how to give up habitual holding patterns. I had then learned to send the messages (directions) to my muscles that would prevent hardening or unnecessary shortening. I then slowly built up the skill in applying these new directions to gradually more challenging movements and situations so that, by the time I attempted to apply them to running, I had improved both my sensory awareness and my ability to sustain directions. Thus, I could: a) sense when I was going wrong; b) do something about it.

When I was out on the road attempting to run again, the first thing I needed to do was to decide *not* to run. Even thinking about running was enough to make me prepare unconsciously to run in my old habitual manner. I needed to pause (inhibit my immediate response to the stimulus) and to project the directions for the optimal functioning of primary control (the head-neck-back relationship), and then continue sending these directions while adding other directions that would get me moving forward.

So, instead of deciding to run, I would allow my neck to be free, let my head go forward and up, let my back lengthen and widen, and only then allow this length to take me forward in an easy loss of balance, knowing that a leg would move under me when needed. I did *not* need to begin by shifting my weight to one leg and reaching out the other to pull myself along.

The pattern of misuse that caused my problem was not unique to running; it was also apparent in my walking and standing, but it might never have caused me discomfort had I not taken up running. This is not because running is 'bad for you', as some would claim, it is because habitual excess effort is increased when running. I hardened my neck and pulled my head back and down when sitting or standing. And when I began to run, I simply did this more ferociously.

I have been running joyously for the past 12 years, have won numerous trophies in races, and have remained mostly injury-free. Often, in a race, I have found myself striving to catch a runner in front of me, and have been able to pause mentally, to give up straining to catch them, and focus instead on my 'use'. I have then seen my breathing slow and have watched myself pass the runner without stress. Whereas in the past it had been necessary to stop running completely to inhibit certain unconscious patterns, it now seems possible to return to a non-doing state in motion. In fact, I do some of my best work on myself while running.

So, while it may be true that running can be bad for you if you use yourself poorly, it is also true that if you use yourself well, running can be very good for you. It is an opportunity to extend yourself into space, to use the full range of movement that a free stride allows, to use your lungs to the fullest, and to allow the ribs to move unimpeded by misplaced effort.

FREEING THE ARMS AND LEGS

The shoulder and hip joints are designed to allow the arms and legs respectively to function independently of the torso. This means, for example, that we can lift or swing our arms without having to shorten the spine. One of the qualities we see in great runners is the head remaining still and the back long (yet dynamic) while the arms and legs do their thing.

An interesting 'test' of independence can be performed in the semi-supine position, with head supported and knees bent. Lift an arm over your head and note whether or not this movement causes any major changes in the neck or back, such as tightening or

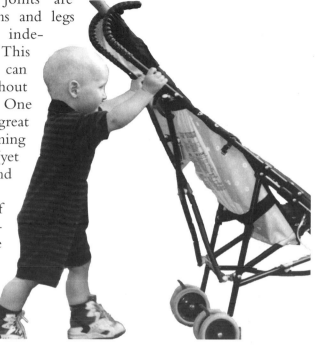

This small boy demonstrates excellent use of 'primary control' while pushing his pram.

twisting. Repeat with the other arm, then try the same procedure with the legs. Gently lift your right foot off the floor and then extend the leg so that it ends up stretched out. Most people find a tendency for the back to compensate when they try this. In fact, it should be possible to lift the leg and stretch it without any tightening of the abdomen or rolling of the pelvis. It took me several months of work before I was able to achieve this, but then I am a slow learner...

The benefit of this procedure is to become aware of the lack of independence between the limbs and the torso, a lack which will be hidden during movement. By learning to reduce it, we should as a result be able to run more freely.

HITTING THE WALL

Like the floor, using a wall can give great feedback about our 'use' – that is, how we organise ourselves both at rest and when we move. This can give the runner insight into what is really happening when s/he runs, and provide the knowledge to make changes and improvements. As Alexander said, 'The things that don't exist are the most difficult to get rid of'.

Stand with your back to the wall, heels about six centimetres (two inches) away from it. Now let yourself lean back against the wall and see which part of your body touches it first.

If your head and/or shoulders touch first, it means that you tend to stand (and run) with the pelvis pushed forward and shoulders leaning back – Fred's 'piss position', you may recall.

If your bum hits first, it means that you tend to stiffen your ankles and legs and reach for the wall with your posterior.

Ideally, your shoulders and buttocks should arrive against the wall at the same time without the back of your head touching at all. If your head is touching, it means that you are tightening your neck and pulling your head back. When a runner 'loses' the ability to cope with the stress of a race, one of the tell-tale signs is that the head gets pulled back into the neck.

So you are now standing with your shoulders and bottom (but not your head) touching the wall. We can use the wall to help orient ourselves, and think of our backs aiming up the wall and towards the ceiling ('back and up'). This thought can be repeated several times until the experience registers kinaes-thetically – that is, until we have a sense of what the words mean. This can be helpful to anyone who tends (and who doesn't?!) to lean a bit too far forward when they run.

Once you get a sense of 'back and up', add the following and see what happens.

Give a thought to releasing the front of the ankle and the back of the knee, and roll your right foot up on to the toe. Did anything change as far as your back is concerned? For example, did your hips come away from the wall? This indicates that your hip joint is a little 'stuck', and when the leg moved forward it pulled your hips with it. This lack of independence shows up in runners who 'sit on the legs'.

The other thing that might have happened is that your right hip collapsed and you sagged a bit. Again, this rock-and-roll shows up among runners in the form of wasted and costly 'lateral displacement of the torso'.

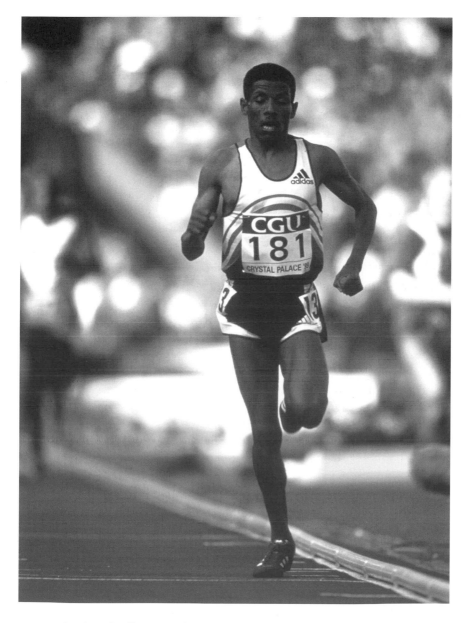

*Haile Gebrsellasie, arguably the world's greatest middle-distance runner,
'going up' while he's looking down.*

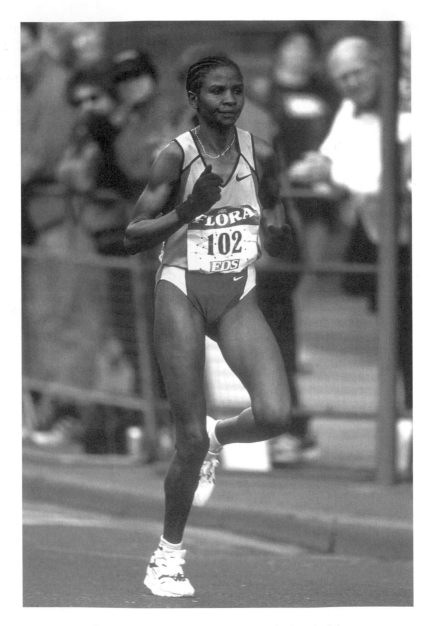

*Joyce Chepchumba demonstrates a style devoid of the
'postural eccentricities' that so bedevil lesser runners.*

If, however, your knee released forward and you rolled gently up on your toe while your spine continued to aim back and up, then you are well on your way to fame and fortune.

Now alternate one foot after the other and see if you can maintain that sense of dynamic stability in your head and torso. Too easy? Try it faster.

When this procedure is done well, it encompasses many of the elements found in good running: a long back which tends to stay up and off the legs, head poised and leading the spine, free ankles and knees for efficient leg movement, balance, independence and co-ordination between the top half of the body and the bottom half, with each part doing its thing in a synchronised and harmonious manner.

Now repeat all this away from the wall! This will increase the demands for balance and freedom, as the wall is no longer there to provide support and feedback.

TAKING THE LUNGE

The lunge looks like the movement performed by a fencer who is trying to skewer an opponent. The leg in front is bent, while the trail leg is straight. *En garde!*

When we practise the lunge, attention is paid to maintaining the relationship between head-neck-back while letting the front knee bend. An emphasis is placed on allowing the head to lead (this is the primary movement) and the leg to bend in response (secondary). This enables the back to 'lengthen and widen', and promotes independence between leg and back.

When this procedure is performed slowly, there is plenty of time to eliminate unnecessary effort and to encourage the correct response to take place. So while your head is leading your spine into length, you can ensure your straight back leg releases and lengthens.

Because the lunge is not that far removed from what we do when we run (except that we don't tip so far forward), this type of stretch can be useful in that we can think the same way 'during the act' and prevent undue shortening in the process. And rather than forcing the front knee to bend any which way, we can encourage it to release out and away over the toe, again with the same action the runner should employ but with a maximum of freedom and awareness. Indeed, having a clear idea of what we would like to happen when we run is one way of improving our running action. Going out and simply hoping that time and experience (and perhaps the good Lord) will help smooth the rough edges is a slow and often painful journey.

While performing the lunge, you may also discover 'postural eccentricities', those cute little habits your mother adored but which drive coaches to distraction. For example, in my experience, many people have no idea how they 'wear their feet': are they pointing straight ahead, at ten to two, or at ten to 12? One thing coaches emphasise in developing a good, efficient, injury-resistant stride is the need to run with feet pointing straight ahead. In contrast, 'toeing-out' adds a certain amount of unnecessary strain on the rest of the body and has serious implications as far as stride length is concerned. A study showed that runners with a size nine foot who toe-out 20 degrees (just one centimetre from straight) lose 16 metres during the course of a mile run. Extend this over a marathon, and it adds up to more than 400 metres – something which could make a considerable difference if you were close to breaking the three-hour barrier.

So if you want to improve your stride, reduce the risk of injuries and better your times without more training, learn and practise the lunge!

THE EYES HAVE IT

No wonder the Kenyans are such great runners – look at their mothers! Kenyan women can carry remarkably heavy loads on their heads, with no loss of poise and, amazingly, no increase in their energy output. Yet they are able to walk for considerable distances over varied terrain without losing their equilibrium. This highlights the important role that head balance plays in movement.

The head, depending on how great a runner you think you are, weighs approximately 4.5 kg (10 lbs). Runners generally like to look down. The connection is obvious.

When asked why they focus on the tarmac, most say it's to avoid stepping in dog mess or to make sure they don't trip on an uneven surface (since most Kenyan women are not walking on Astroturf we must wonder how they manage). Both reasons have some validity. Indeed, going for a little jog recently in Paris, I found completing the run unscathed presented quite a challenge!

There is no reason why a runner can't or shouldn't survey the path – especially when they balance their head freely. But what happens in practice is that runners make looking down the rule and looking ahead the exception. Now if you ask someone to leave their head still while looking first to the right and then to the left, you will notice a tendency for the person's head to follow the movement of their eyes. And when it comes to looking down, most people like to tilt the head from the base of the neck in order to see what's coming. You can imagine what would happen to the jug of water on our Kenyan woman's head if she did this every time a rock or branch loomed in her path…

So what effect does looking down have on the runner?

• **Runners who look down tend to run heavier.** When I ask runners to rate their foot impact on the ground on a scale from 1-10 (light to heavy), first when looking down and then when gazing into the distance, they invariably rate impact as being lighter when they look ahead.

'Running heavy' is associated with various complaints, from foot, shin and leg problems to the oft-heard warning: 'Running jars your spine'. I remember one runner I worked with who you could hear hitting the ground enthusiastically as he went along. When asked if he was aware how hard he landed, he said that he was – but it was much better than before. When asked to elaborate, he recounted how, two-thirds of the way through a 30k race, he started to feel the pain of his efforts. So in a bid to maintain his pace he consciously started to drive his feet into the ground – as he put it, to 'pound through the pain'. The result was that he pounded his way into a stress fracture which kept him sidelined for six months.

• **Neck and shoulder pain.** As an experiment, try holding a 4.5 kg (10 lbs) weight out in front of you for a while. It takes a lot of effort. When the head is tilted forward from the base of the neck, it puts tremendous strain on the neck and shoulders – which have to work very hard to keep the head from falling off and hitting the ground. This problem is compounded when the runner, in an effort to see ahead, looks up by pulling the head back and increasing the curve and strain on the neck and spine. This tendency can lead to the development of a hump at the base of the neck.

• **Looking down encourages runners to lean forward and to shorten the front of their bodies.** In an article in *Runner's World* entitled 'Posture Perfect', Tim Galloway points out that runners who lean too far forward tend to cut an inch off their stride – which at a ten-minute-mile pace would add more than seven minutes to their marathon time. He also points out that runners who lean forward and shorten tend to have more difficulty breathing, something most runners would surely like to minimise!

In contrast, looking ahead gives the brain sufficient lag time to see what's coming up, and tell the feet what to avoid and how to adjust. This is particularly important for runners who train on uneven surfaces – or just wish to avoid the dog shit…

BEARING ARMS

I'm always amazed at how many armless runners I see out there. By armless, I'm referring to the familiar sight of runners plodding along with their arms held stiffly and stuck to their sides. What little movement there is often involves the shoulders, so that the whole torso sways from side to side. Running in this way is like driving with the handbrake on. It can be done, but you are always working against yourself.

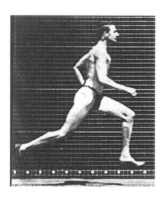 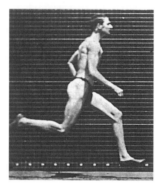 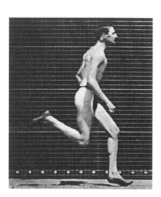

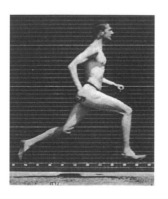 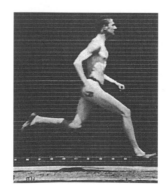 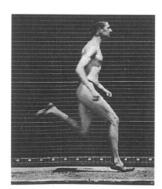

Contrast this with the arm movement we see on many top runners: elbows bent at 90 degrees, wrists neither floppy nor rigid, and the arms moving back-wards and forwards, sometimes coming slightly across the body but with very little sway in the torso. When the arms are used in a co-ordinated and rhythmic fashion, they are a wonderful source of power and energy as well as balancing the movement of the legs. How much does a runner lose by not taking advantage?

Try this simple experiment to get a sense of how much you may be robbing yourself. First, find a small hill 30-50 metres long. Now hook your thumbs in the top of your shorts and then run up the hill. Notice how much energy this takes and how hard the legs have to work. Then return to the bottom of the hill and this time start pumping your arms like a sprinter and run up the hill for a second time. Which was easier? If you are like many runners, you will find the latter experience much more agreeable.

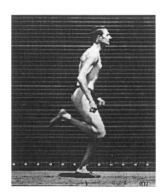
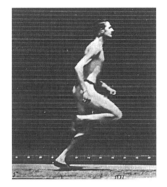
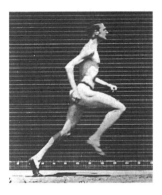

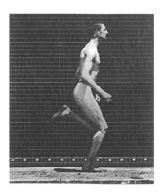

This sequence, and two later in the book, come from The Human Figure in Motion *by Eadweard Muybridge (1830-1904), the British artist, inventor and photographer who is often hailed as the 'Father of Motion Pictures'. During the 1850s, Muybridge created a device he called a zoopraxiscope to project single sequential images and give the illusion of movement. While it is a matter of conjecture whether he helped inspire Thomas Edison to begin his experiments in motion photography, Muybridge certainly proved for the first time that all four hooves leave the ground when a horse trots. In 1884-85 he began photographing hundreds of ordinary people in an attempt to catalogue the diversity of human motion against a fixed grid: this runner, for example, is 'armless', depriving himself of the energy that comes from using the arms in a more powerful and co-ordinated manner.*

A TEACHER'S EXPERIENCE – MICK

I hadn't run in any consistent way since I left school more than 20 years ago, but I decided I needed to improve my fitness and struggled, huffing and puffing, round the local park for the first six weeks. As an Alexander Technique teacher, I was aware of the need to keep my direction and avoid inappropriate effort. However, a running lesson with Malcolm Balk changed my whole understanding of running and has turned it into an experience I now look forward to and enjoy.

There were several key points which dramatically changed my running style. First, there was the use of my eyes. My tendency to look down at the ground in front of me was literally taking me down. Learning to scan the middle distance made a tangible difference to my sense of length and to the heaviness of my footfall. I had been allowing my eyes to drag my head forward and down, bringing my neck with it and upsetting the poise of my head–neck–back relationship. This, in turn, affected the way I used my legs. They struggled to keep up with me as I fell or pulled myself forward and down onto the ground.

My poor understanding of 'how' to run compounded the problems further. I knew that I did not want to use *unnecessary* effort, but I was confusing this with *appropriate* effort from the arms and legs. I had always held my arms steady by my sides as I ran. This, I erroneously believed, would help me conserve energy. Malcolm showed that by using the arms properly, I could actually decrease the effort I used in my legs and in an overall sense improve my 'use' when running. By actively bringing back my arms with elbows bent, my legs were more easily activated. I could also use the speed of the arm movement to control my pace and determine how fast I ran. This was another revelation, and made a dramatic difference to both my running style and my subjective experience.

By using my arms appropriately, it felt like my legs were automatically activated to the degree necessary to the task. The other major difference when I used my arms was that it felt like my whole torso was lifted off my legs. This gave my legs more space and time to swing forward under me, and offer support at the appropriate phase of the running cycle. Previously they had been lagging behind, and the combination of the way I used my eyes and did not use my legs was making it impossible for my legs to do anything other than struggle to try and keep up.

As I learned to keep my length and 'stay off my legs', I was able to use my legs to better effect. Instead of trailing behind, I had actively to lift my knees more in order to get my legs in synch with my arms and back.

As my understanding of good running technique improved, my style changed dramatically and running became the pleasure that it is today. At first, the new style felt odd. I thought that anyone watching me would see a cartoon caricature of a runner. I especially felt that I was lifting my knees too high, but this was in comparison to my old tendency to let them trail behind me too much. I soon began to feel like a well-oiled machine, where my legs act as a suspension system which supports me. Running has now become a co-ordinated activity, where appropriate effort in each part combines to create optimal use of the whole structure.

FAST AND LOOSE

Another experiment I call 'changing gears' involves what track athletes know as accelerations, usually of 100 metres. The runner starts slowly and gradually increases the pace up to 80-90 per cent of top speed before easing off over the last 20 metres. These are used to warm up and get used to running at a faster pace.

First, increase speed by just moving your legs faster. Note how much effort this takes. You may also notice that you throw your head back and tighten your shoulders. Now try accelerating a second time by letting the arms lead and the legs follow. This means that each time you change gears from first to fourth (for those of you who can't afford a Porsche, this is your chance to create a little Porsche energy), you simply allow the arms to move more quickly in an ever increasing arc and let your legs follow suit. During this procedure, the head should remain lightly poised on top of the spine and the shoulders stay nice and wide.

No? Then you are probably trying too hard to get it right. Begin again and build up gradually, not worrying about how fast you go at first. You can also reverse the process if you have space, going from fourth to first simply by slowing and reducing the movement of the arms without leaning backwards or shortening ('running small').

Most runners find this way of 'changing gears' is easier, involves less effort and is much more fun!

STATE OF INDEPENDENCE

Running consists of putting one leg in front of the other. This simple act can be performed in many different ways, some better than others. To help us understand what differentiates 'good' running from the rest, we need to study the concepts of 'independence' and 'dynamic stability'.

Independence is the ability to move one bit of our body without having to move everything else. Anyone who has ever had a crick in their neck and has needed to turn their whole body in order to see over their shoulder knows its value. We have already discussed the consequences of a lack of independence between the eyes and the head. However, a co-ordinated activity like running also requires a certain degree of independence of the legs from the torso, the arms from the torso, and the head from the neck. Here are three ways to achieve this.

The typical pattern involves 'posturing oneself' by tightening the torso so that it is held in place with a lot of muscular tension. The common advice given in running magazines and books, and by many doctors and physiotherapists, is to develop the abdominal and back muscles to 'support' the torso. Sometimes additional corrective measures are recommended, such as tilting the pelvis or tucking the chin.

The problem with this approach is that it tends to pull things towards each other – as in the case of the sit-up, where the ribs are pulled towards the pelvis; the pelvic tilt, which pushes the pelvis into the legs; and the chin tuck, which pulls the head into the neck. A tendency to tighten or fix has at least three negative effects: it makes it harder to breathe, it makes it harder to move, and it makes us less aware of what may be going on in our bodies.

A second tendency is for runners to 'collapse' – not just after finishing a tough race or workout, but during the act of running itself. It's debatable whether this is based on the idea that running is a leg activity so we can let the rest of the body take a breather, a faulty concept of 'running relaxed', or a lack of awareness regarding the inter-relation of the legs and torso. Whatever the reason, the result

Lengthening doesn't necessarily have to be vertical, as this small girl demonstrates.

is the same: independence and potential are reduced, and more effort and energy are required.

The third option is familiar to most Alexandrians and some runners. Stability in the torso, or the head–neck–back relationship, is dynamic in nature, with the head remaining poised on top of the spine and the back tending to lengthen and widen. The result is a state of dynamic stability, characterised by expansion of the whole body framework rather than contraction.

RUNNING TALL

Most, though by no means all, running coaches extol the value and importance of 'running tall' in order to achieve optimal performance. In the aforementioned 'Posture Perfect' article, Tim Galloway lists ten benefits of running with good posture. These include running more easily, suffering fewer injuries and breathing more efficiently.

Coaches try different means to encourage runners into this state. Two examples from Galloway's article include the advice of the great New Zealand coach Arthur Lydiard, who suggests that we imagine a pulley attached to our breastbone, that a rope runs through it to the top of a small building a block away, and that the rope is pulling you towards the top of the building as a way of helping you to lift your chest as you run. Galloway himself proposes that we think of ourselves suspended like puppets from a thread attached to our heads.

As runners, we are also urged to tuck the pelvis under, to belly-breathe, and so on. Most of this advice, while well intentioned, causes as many problems as it attempts to solve. Here is an example of this.

In western society, it is sad but true that the slump is much more the norm than the beautifully lengthened back of the tribesman or woman. In my experience as an Alexandrian over the past 20 years, it is extremely rare to find someone who, when asked to stand at full height, does not immediately assume some variation on a military stance: the neck is tightened and the head pulled into the spine, causing it to compress, while the chest is raised, causing the lower back to tighten and hollow and the knees and legs to stiffen. This 'posture' requires considerable effort to maintain. Runners by nature are a persistent lot and many, to their detriment, will try to incorporate some variation of this into their running, kilometre after kilometre. The result is a far cry from the natural, efficient poise we are seeking.

BREATHING

Over the years I have heard a lot of different suggestions about how to breathe when you run. First of all, I must say that I have always thought it a good idea to breathe when running as it helps to keep that unsightly bluish tint out of the cheeks!

Alexander was known in the early part of his career as the 'Breathing Man' because he was able to help people improve in this area. From his personal experience and that of helping others, he concluded that you could not improve breathing without improving a person's 'use'.

'I learned from these experiences,' he wrote, 'that I could not enable my pupils to control the functioning of their organs, systems or reflexes directly, but that by teaching them to employ consciously the primary control of their use I could put them in command of the means whereby their functioning generally can be indirectly controlled.'

One thing you often read in running magazines and books on the subject is that runners should 'belly breathe'. The reasons for this advice are a) to counteract the bad habit of pulling the belly in when inhaling (thereby interfering with the natural movement of the diaphragm) and b) to use more lung capacity than one would by simply breathing with the chest. Taken at face value, this seems like reasonable advice which should be simple enough to carry out – enabling a runner to reap the benefits. But hold on there, not so fast!

An example from my own experience highlights the danger of trying to improve breathing directly. After reading about the benefits of belly breathing back in the 1970s, I dutifully put it into practice mile after mile during preparation for various marathons. Along the way, I also developed a chronic ache in my lower back. It wasn't until I got into the Alexander Technique in the early '80s that I made the connection between the way I was belly breathing and the pain I was suffering. I realised that in pushing my abdomen out with every inhalation (20 or so times per minute), I was arching my lower back and creating strain in that area in the process.

This was further exacerbated by clinging to another piece of advice you often hear: that you must strengthen (in other words, tighten) the abdominal muscles to avoid back problems. So there I was, trying to push my belly out against those tight abs – absolutely ludicrous, but not unusual in the world of the quick fix. Just to see what I'm talking about, try pushing out your belly when you inhale and see if you don't feel your lower back tighten or arch.

Now, just for laughs, tighten your stomach and try to push it out when inhaling. Notice anything else getting involved, like your neck and shoulders?

A quick anatomical point here: the bottom of the front of the lungs is about seven centimetres (three inches) below the nipple. In other words, there isn't any way possible of getting air into the abdomen, short of being shot! So the very term 'belly breathing' is easily open to mis-interpretation. When the diaphragm (the breathing muscle) descends during an in-breath, it pushes down on the organs and other contents of the abdominal cavity, causing the cavity to expand if we allow it to do so. Also note that the whole torso, including the back, expands during the in-breath, not just the abdomen. By trying to push the abdomen out, you may well be preventing the rest of your torso from participating in the movement of breathing as it was designed to do – particularly the rib cage.

One of the fundamental differences between the Alexander Technique and other approaches can be summarised thus: if there is something wrong, don't 'do the opposite', the usual 'cure' for most problems, but find out what it is and stop it. This implies more of an 'undoing' rather than adding on another layer of 'doing'. Instead of pushing the belly out to prevent it from tightening during inhalation, you need to learn to release it during this phase of breathing. Now, in my experience it is really hard to tighten your abdomen (to support the back) and release at the same time (in order to breathe)! However, if you learn to lengthen and widen your torso as you run, your abdomen will naturally respond to the rhythm of your breathing as well as providing whatever other support is required. In fact, as I've mentioned, it isn't just your abdomen that moves when you breathe, but your back also expands in response to the movement of the diaphragm.

What prevents this from happening? The major culprit is 'pulling down'. When we shorten ourselves, we get in the way and have to compensate by raising the shoulders, arching the back or lifting the sternum. Much better to prevent the interference than add on some new 'improvement'.

The benefits of breathing through the nose are well-known. One of the procedures used in Alexander Technique, the 'whispered ah', encourages us to allow inhalation through the nose. For many years as a runner, I never thought of breathing in this way. In fact, I thought it would be impossible. Well, I was wrong!

In his book, *Mind, Body and Sport*, John Douilliard describes a novel approach to breathing when running. He suggests that we should learn to breathe through the nose, rather than through the mouth as is more common. He points out that mouth breathing has several limitations: it is associated with hyperventilation; it tends to be shallower; and it stimulates the parasympathetic nervous system which results in a 'flight or fight' response. This may be useful when avoiding a vicious dog, but is hardly conducive to the sense of release and flow we are seeking on a run. Breathing through the nose, according to Douillard's research, is what most animals do in their natural state, except under stress (such as when being hunted). It allows air to be filtered, moistened and warmed; it is generally deeper, meaning more oxygen is made available to our working muscles; and it tends to stimulate the sympathetic nervous system which helps calm us down. There is another interesting effect: nose breathing usually helps to lower the heart rate.

When I first tried to breathe through my nose, I found myself constantly panicking and having to gasp in some air through my mouth. I needed to slow down, something which was very difficult for a semi-reformed 'end-gainer' – oops, I mean competitive runner! – like myself. For some weeks, I found myself letting runners whom I would normally 'thrash' pass me by and disappear into the distance. This was initially quite hard on my running ego, as I had always maintained a certain status on my regular training route up Mount Royal. But the funny thing was that running started to feel less like an obligation or duty and more like something I was once again beginning to enjoy. It made me realise that I had fallen into the competitive runner's trap of always pushing myself, even when it wasn't necessary.

As I continued the nose-breathing experiments on easy runs, I gradually discovered that my pace was increasing but my heart rate was staying low. As a result, running started to feel less stressful. Eventually, I could run at my 'normal' easy pace and maintain nose breathing. This translated into an ability to race with less stress and reduce the cramping I sometimes suffered. But a note of caution here: one can easily put a lot of unnecessary effort into nose breathing, which will reduce any benefit you might gain from the practice. And two common habits which should be avoided are sniffing and pulling the head back.

One of the ways to avoid 'end-gaining' during a run, an example of which could be running faster than you'd planned, is to pay attention to your breathing rate. The general rule of thumb for beginners on an easy run is to go at a speed at which you can maintain a conversation. This will help the runner stay within his or her aerobic limits and not go into oxygen debt. Jack Daniels notes that most élite middle- and long-distance runners race at what he calls a 2-2 pace. That is, they either breathe in or breathe out every two steps, as in: right (inhale), left, right (exhale), left and so on. Slower-paced runs are carried out at a 3-3 or a 4-4 rhythm. Paying attention to breathing rate can help the runner to avoid over-training. As Daniels points out, 'If 3-3 does not provide you with enough air on an easy run, then it's not an easy run. Slow down to where 3-3 is comfortable'.

Finally, it is important to remember that it is impossible to improve your breathing without improving your 'use'. As Patrick Macdonald points out in his book, *The Alexander Technique As I See It*: 'If you allow your ribs to move, as nature intended, you will breathe properly. What you have to learn is to let them move.' Let is the operative word. Most people, particularly athletes or those who have done breathing exercises, hold their ribs very fixed. There is a way of freeing the ribs but it is not specifically for the ribs. It involves a change in the head-neck-back relationship and often, indeed, a change in the whole structure of the torso.

WALKING AND RUNNING

When considering walking, the first thought must be to gain one's full height. Having established and engaged the conscious directions for this, the upright body is now at its maximum precariousness being fully alive and poised. Minimal forward inclination will start the process of walking, whereby one finds oneself in effect 'falling upwards' as one travels forwards. Once walking is underway, the back remains 'back and up' to 'come up off the legs', so that the legs move freely. This method, simple as it may appear, is not, however, the one usually adopted. Nearly everyone employs physical tension in such a way that there is a tendency to shorten the spine and legs, by pressing down through the floor instead of lightening that pressure by lengthening the body and easing forward and up to move lightly and freely.

It is possible to move in many different ways, as anyone observing a local fun run will attest. Sometimes the variations can be pretty funny, although they are usually not intended as such. I am assuming that the reason you are reading this book is not to develop the tragi-comic aspects of your stride, but to change, reduce or eliminate them. In his article 'Together We Walk', Walton L White points out that some ways of walking (and, by extension, running) are better than others: 'Some ways are basic patterns evolution worked out for us long ago; others are distortions we have imposed on these basic patterns, often with an added tax of unnecessary effort. We can become so accustomed to paying this added tax that we don't recognise it as such and take it as part of the original price.'

He goes on: 'There's a big difference in the effort I make during walking when I merely extend my body upward over my foot and when I try to push the ground down and back away from me. In the first instance I just move my body away from the ground; in the second, I am trying to move the whole planet away from me. It shouldn't surprise anyone, however, that it takes more effort to push the planet than to push my body.'

Be it walking, running or any other form of movement, one of the benefits of learning the Alexander Technique is that it can help you become more sensitive about how you 'put the brakes on' when you move. You start to learn how to 'flow', how to get out of the way and let 'it' move you. In *The Alexander Technique As I See It*, Patrick Macdonald describes this phenomenon: 'When a pupil is capable of acting without interfering with the primary control, or perhaps I should say with only slight interfering, the actionless activity that is going on in the body modifies the physical activity and brings it into harmony with itself, so that the physical activity grows out of the non-doing of the primary control. To the trained eye, it is a great pleasure to watch anyone whose physical actions are determined in this way.'

GOING INTO MOVEMENT

For many people, the transition from the 'resting state' to running represents their greatest hurdle! In other words, how to get off the couch and out of the front door...

Sadly, the following procedure is not designed to help the terminally idle, but focuses instead on what happens in the time between the decision to take a step and the moment when you actually take it.

Stand in front of a mirror or reflective window with your feet fairly close together. Take a step forward and note the amount of sway. To make this even more fun, ask a friend to watch and see if they can guess which foot you are going to step with before you actually move. Most people telegraph their intention by leaning over to one side – the left side if they are going to step

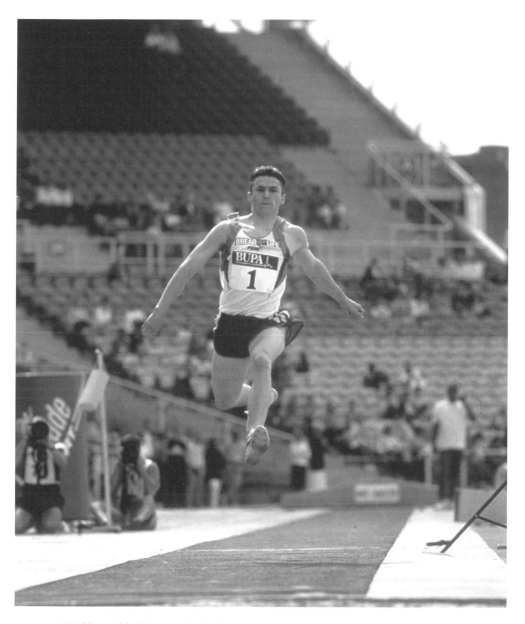

World record-holder Jonathan Edwards in action: complex events like the triple jump require athletes to 'stretch their envelope' every time they train and compete.

with the right foot. The question that needs to be asked is, 'Why does this happen and what does it mean for us as runners?' In Alexander terms, what it means is that we have forgotten to release and rise to our full height as we make to step.

The lean is related to our need to balance ourselves. The desire not to land on our butt is very strong and, for the most part, unconscious. Whenever we feel out of balance, a little alarm bell goes off in the form of what Alexander called a 'fear reflex' and the result is that we stiffen ourselves. This is why we lean: we are simply trying not to fall over.

The significance of this for runners is that leaning from side to side is simply wasteful and places added stress on the side that's being leaned on. But the good news is that it's not necessary. Just like you can learn to lift one leg off the ground and not shift everything over to the other side like an unbalanced beanbag chair, you can also learn to minimise this tendency when you run. And one of the best times by far to learn this skill is when you go into motion.

Argument overheard in workshop why this is impossible: 'If I lift up my right leg, I have to shift everything over to the left. Where else is it going to go?' – followed by a massive lean to the left.

Clever answer: 'Rather than thinking of weight going from side to side, think of it going up and down or forwards and backwards – and maybe even both at the same time!'

There are other things to think about when taking a step. Do you tighten or release into motion: do you flow up into a movement, or start things off with a little contractive jerk? It's like learning to drive a car with a clutch. Do you want to pop it, or ease it up so that the transition from stop to go is barely perceptible?

Here's another clever question: what leads the movement? Obviously the head leads, but what is the sequence after that? Some people might say the hip, others the knee, and both are good guesses. In fact it is the knee, but first the ankle needs to release. It's very hard to let the ankle bend if it's stiff or held; release it and the knee is very happy to follow suit.

When you are out for a walk and have to stop for some reason, see how smooth you can make that first step. Keep breathing, and try to iron out the leaning, shoving, lurching and jerking as you begin to move by releasing your neck, lengthening yourself and 'falling up' into it. You are now well on your way to becoming a 'conscious runner'.

STRETCHING YOUR ENVELOPE

Human beings are creatures of habit, and runners tend always to go at the same pace. Once a certain proficiency and fitness level are achieved, we often chug along on automatic pilot. This can vary from the positively pedestrian to sub-six minute miles, depending on our level.

This can be a good thing in that it allows us to muse, spectate or carry on a conversation without having to attend to the physical and technical requirements of moving. But the trouble with always running at the same pace is that it starts to become mechanical and unconscious. Bad habits become ingrained and disappear into the recesses of awareness. We are no longer in touch with ourselves. If we all ran like Kenyans, maybe this wouldn't be such a big deal – but we don't. In order that we continue to enjoy our activity by avoiding injury and boredom, we need to reconnect. One way to do this is to 'stretch the envelope' and do something a little different. Not only will this get your attention, it will make you a better runner.

Here are two examples aimed at the extremes of the running continuum. For the slower folks who are sometimes called joggers, you need to change gear occasionally. It's not enough just to plod along for 30 minutes, zoning out with your Walkman. There are heights of enjoyment you will never experience in that mode. For ten minutes of your run, try picking up the pace a little maybe from one lamp post to the next. Then go back to your normal speed for a pole or two, then repeat. And continue like this for the next five to ten minutes. It isn't a question of exhausting yourself, even though your breathing will quicken and you may feel initially that you are overdoing it: it's causing you to wake up and pay attention to what's going on, getting you to reconnect with the moment, to notice how you are reacting to the stimulus, and thereby giving you an opportunity to practise 'thinking in activity'. What at first seems difficult, unnecessary or even an irritation will become a source of interest and enjoyment.

For faster runners, those who think going at anything less than a mile pace of 6 min 30 secs is an act of cowardice and wimpishness, try running a couple of minutes slower but with perfect form. Same leg cadence, same movement with the arms and legs although in a slightly reduced form – in other words, a miniature version of your normal long, flowing stride. Many advanced runners' form tends to deteriorate drastically when they are just out for an easy run or in their warm-up/cool-down phase before or after a race.

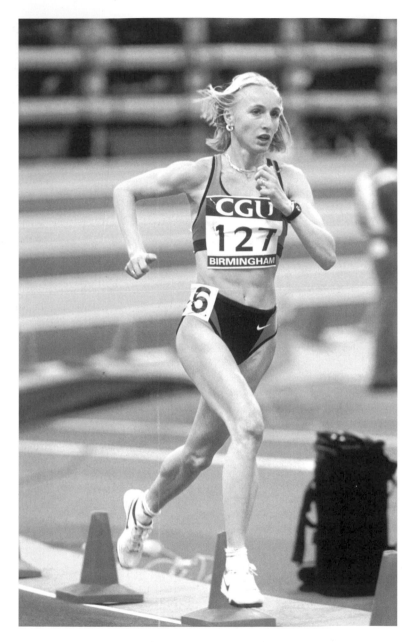

Gabriella Szabo demonstrates a perfect 'double-spiral' pattern – see opposite.

Here is a quotation from a runner I used to nag about paying attention to his stride. Some years after he had moved on to bigger and better things, I received the following note describing his latest thoughts on form: 'The running stride must be mechanically sound at all times. Often the slow gait of an easy run is entirely inappropriate training for the body. You lean back, run on the heels and use a cadence that programs the mind and body for a slower turnover. You should be using race-cadence in order to condition muscle elasticity and to optimise and harmonise your frequency in preparation for race conditions.

'This represents a radical change from the way I've always run. I've detected some horrendously inefficient tendencies in my stride: heel striking, no toe drive, dropping the arms, head and shoulders thrown back. And so I have been emphasising two crucial points during workouts and easy runs: a) lead with the upper body; b) bounce off the toes.'

He goes on to add that he thinks Gabriella Szabo's form is ideal, so during his easy runs he imagines he's a 40 kg Romanian woman. He has managed at 85 kg to run 3 min 49 secs for 1,500 and 2 hr 31 mins for the marathon!

LET'S TWIST AGAIN

During all my years of looking at running through an Alexandrian lens, I had advocated leaving the trunk still while the arms moved independently from the shoulder joint. I did this in spite of what I had observed in many great runners: that they allow their shoulders to rotate slightly around the spine with each swing of the arm. I had always thought this wasteful and unnecessary. However, if some of the best athletes in the world move in this fashion, then it was surely time for me to reconsider my definition of efficient running.

I recently watched Paul Collins, an Alexander Technique teacher and age-group ultra-distance world record-holder, in a video he made before his death. In this film, he explained our ability to rotate in what he called a 'double spiral' pattern. The body, he insisted, has a natural tendency to turn around the spine if it is not held stiffly in place. A child reaching for a toy will demonstrate this pattern beautifully. You might notice the same thing when shaking hands.

This rotation or spiral is balanced by a counter-rotation in the hips, so that when the left knee goes forward (hips thus spiralling to the right) it is balanced by the right arm (upper torso spiralling to the left). I believe that the action of the spirals is what connects the movement of the arms to that of the legs in running. This also helps to explain what Percy Cerutty meant by running 'on the legs not with the legs'. Some of the ways we prevent this natural movement are by 'postural fixations', such as carrying things in the arms or pulling down when we sit slumped in front of a computer.

The spiralling action is facilitated by the atlanto-occipital joint in the neck, which enables us to turn our head freely without having to move the shoulders. It also allows us to rotate the shoulders and torso while the head remains still and poised. Without this joint, every time our bodies turned the head would be obliged to follow, like someone with a stiff neck or an amateur shoplifter.

Finally, the spiralling activity we see in so many top athletes seems to work best when the runner's spine is at its optimal length – in other words, s/he is 'running tall'.

MY STORY – DOUG

At the start of my first Alexander Technique and running course in 1995, all the participants told each other why they were there. I said: 'I used to enjoy running but I've spoiled the pleasure by a habit of beating up on myself. I'd like to stop that.' I tend to take things too seriously.

When I joined Thames Valley Harriers in London, I started running a lot more, improved quickly and made the team for the UK cross-country championships. I then had several unplanned months off. Starting up again, I never rediscovered my initial enthusiasm: I wasn't physically injured and I didn't know why I had stopped running. Only when I read my training log sometime later did I see that I'd set myself some absurdly over-ambitious targets to increase my speed. I had also begun resenting the intrusion of running into the rest of my life. My competitiveness had spoiled the fun of it.

Now, if I ask myself: 'Why should I bother going out to run?', the answer is: 'Because it will be pleasant and interesting. And nice afterwards, too.' Before, the answer would have been: 'Well, I won't enjoy the actual running but I'll be glad afterwards that I did it.' So it's easier for me to feel motivated to run these days!

My habit had almost always been to over-train then quit. I'm now establishing a new habit of working more easily and more consistently. I feel I've so far got a rather tenuous hold on the understanding that I shouldn't run too often or too hard for my level of fitness. I don't yet want to go back into a situation (like club membership) where there will be additional temptations to return to my over-training habit (perhaps in order to beat club mates, or to see short-term gains).

Interestingly, this understanding has also helped my professional life. I'm a freelance accountant and my pattern of work as an employee was the same as it was as a running club member: absurd over-ambition alternating with disenchantment. This was baffling at the time but, with hindsight, I know clearly was the result of overdoing things. I now work independently instead and, like my running, it's sustainable, interesting and fun.

There have been other unexpected benefits. Recently I walked into an Underground station and found myself facing a dense crowd of people hurrying in the opposite direction. For the first time in my life, I passed calmly and easily between them. It was very clear where I should walk and there was no bumping or conflict. Somehow I was able to gauge the crowd's various positions, directions and speeds, related them to my own, and adjusted without any bother. Initially, this ease and sharpened perception lasts only a few minutes or hours after working with a teacher. But gradually, more of it stays with you – and you can regain it by working on your own as well.

Some runners are too floppy, while others drive themselves too hard. While floppy people don't apply enough gas, I'm in the 'too hard' group and have become aware that when I thought I was moving full speed ahead I was unwittingly 'driving with the brakes on'. Through the Technique, I've learned how to release the brakes of excess tension and irrelevant movement.

This is just common sense, isn't it? It only becomes common sense once you've noticed what you're doing in the first place. In my own running I had – step by step – reached an understanding that was a long way from everyday common sense and it went something like this: 'If it hurts, keep going; if you don't want to do it, do it anyway'. So I have needed a lot of help to regain a more sensitive (and sensible) appreciation of what I do with myself when I run.

The problem for most of us trying to improve our running form by reading books is that we can't sense very well either what we're currently doing, or the improved form we're trying to achieve. But if you want to explore the ideas in these pages you will certainly need a teacher to help you perceive what you can't see and to appreciate the connections between things which you can't yet feel are connected. I've found that it's not a matter of replacing one unconscious habit with another learned and ultimately unthinking habit. It's about thinking all the time and thinking in a way that releases your power and movement, rather than blocking it.

Your teacher will also encourage you to notice, experiment and play in your running. S/he will discourage you from fixating on short-term gains, times and distances. Other ways of understanding and working with running will be respected. I needed this curious, but non-judgmental, interest in order to perceive more about my current state and its many subtle connections. Once you appreciate more fully where you are now, you can choose your next steps. And the whole process becomes very interesting. On the other hand, if you remain harshly self-critical, you will continue to block your perceptions in order to avoid the related self-criticism.

The work should enable you to observe, react, think and adjust during your run. You will no longer be limited to forming an initial plan and then hanging on to it grimly through the pain barrier.

I enjoy running a lot more since I have:

• Reminded myself why I do it – namely, for pleasure.

• Stopped looking for, or anticipating, side-benefits.

• Stopped planning to run particular distances or times, or on specific days.

• Walked the first bit, rather than started to run straight away.

• Reminded myself during runs: 'The most important thing about this run is that I should finish it wanting to start the next one'.

• Reminded myself, if finding I'm looking forward to the end of a run: 'You don't sing a song, or do a run, to get to the end'.

• Attended to the need to stay relaxed or relax more, rather than driving on. This is a point confirmed by expert race commentators who say things like: 'If she can avoid stiffening up, she'll win', or 'He's got a finish, but he just can't let it out'.

• Looked where I'm going, further up the route in the distance, not just immediately in front of me.

TECHNIQUE, PROCEDURES AND THE MEANING OF LIFE

For those runners among you who have joined a 'serious' club or team, you will probably be asked/required by your coach to perform some drills as part of your training. This is not necessarily a bad thing. Drills and other conditioning aids are used in most sports; in a way, they're like scales and arpeggios in music. They help an athlete warm up, develop a kinaesthetic picture of the correct stride pattern, and improve running technique.

Drills can also work against the runner, by reinforcing existing patterns of poor co-ordination and misuse. Alexander addressed this issue: 'A person who learns to work to a principle in doing one exercise will have learned to do all exercises,' he wrote, 'but the person who learns just "to do an exercise" will most assuredly have to go on learning to do exercises *ad infinitum*.' Here are some ways in which the Alexandrian runner can put drills to good use:

• **As a stimulus for greater co-ordination.** Most drills will make it harder to maintain a state of general co-ordination. For example, it is more difficult to run lifting your knees high than to walk. However, this increase in difficulty can also inspire you to greater heights of co-ordination: learning to do hard things well can help you do easy things better.

You can also use drills to challenge your powers of co-ordination. Alexander used his 'positions of mechanical advantage' to encourage better breathing and overall co-ordination: we've already looked at some of them in detail. I have developed several procedures and adapted others from the coaching repertoire which serve a similar purpose. For example, in order to strengthen a runner's head-neck-back relationship, I will gently challenge them to run slowly up a hill for ten metres, moving arms and legs in a kind of march. This is similar to what an Alexander Technique teacher might do in a private lesson when leaning a pupil slightly backwards off the vertical while sitting in a chair. This puts greater demands on the pupil to maintain length and not tighten the neck or allow the head to pull back. The typical reaction to this stimulus is to tighten the stomach muscles and hold oneself up. By inhibiting this response and continuing the direction to release and lengthen, the pupil will get a much stronger sense of the back offering support than when sitting vertically.

When a runner is asked to run slowly uphill with the knees springing up in front, the stimulus of going uphill in such a fashion may cause them suddenly to forget the back and start to focus on the legs. The whole experience then

107

becomes much more difficult on every level, and may quickly degenerate into a test of strength and endurance. This is not what needs to happen. When the runner stays with his/her back and continues to lengthen, the result is one of effortlessness and flow.

I have witnessed many non-runners perform this procedure and be absolutely astonished to find themselves at the top of a 40-metre hill with none of their expected sense of fatigue – in fact, not even out of breath! It was as though the back, not the legs, took them upwards.

I tried this procedure of 'running with the back' with a fellow teacher and then had him run on level ground. He found the experience so different from what he was used to that he ended up racing around the field like a kid with a new toy. Later, he said 'it was like I found my internal spring'.

• **To improve your ability consciously to inhibit by treating the request to do a drill as a provocation for you to forget your primary directions and start end-gaining.** What a mouthful! What I'm trying to suggest here is that you 'act as if' your coach is deliberately trying to put you wrong! As if he or she is trying to make you stiffen your neck, arch your back and try too hard. Your job is to resist these efforts.

Both as an Alexander Technique teacher and an athletics coach, I spend a fair amount of time trying to help people develop the kind of attitude that is conducive to learning. I know how hard it is with myself not to fall into the trap of becoming mechanical and mindless. My wife will jolt me back to reality sometimes when she nicely points out that I've just gone and done what I told her I would change (I'm pretty good with putting the toilet seat down but I like to leave my running gear on the floor!).

One of the ways I might do this would be to tell a runner that they're looking a bit slow and weak today . . . just before I ask them to accelerate over the last 100 metres of a 1,000-metre repeat. Good runners can make the transition from medium to fast smoothly and efficiently. Frank Shorter wrote of the great Finnish runner, Lasse Viren: 'He had a very smooth stride that essentially did not change as he accelerated in the final laps. Unlike most distance runners, he did not switch to a sprinter's gait in a furious drive to the finish. Somehow he was able to maintain his form... and simply run faster. It was all rpm – his leg rate quickened, which made his speed deceptive. It was something to see.' Viren is the only athlete to win the 5,000 and 10,000 metres at two Olympic Games: 1972 and 1976.

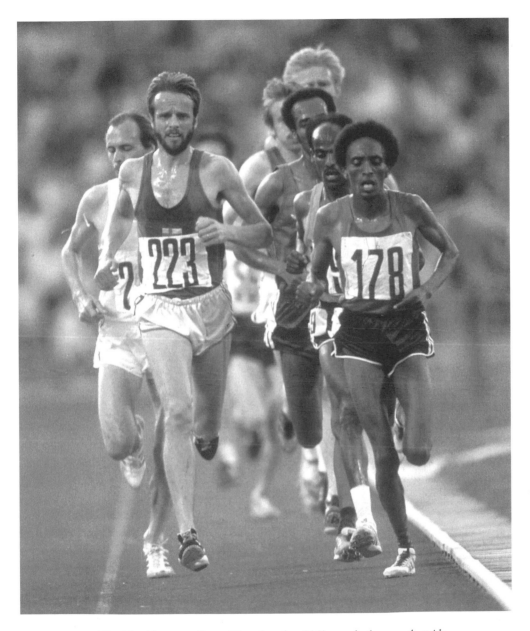

The Finnish runner Lasse Viren (number 223) reveals the smooth stride and good form that can make speed deceptive.

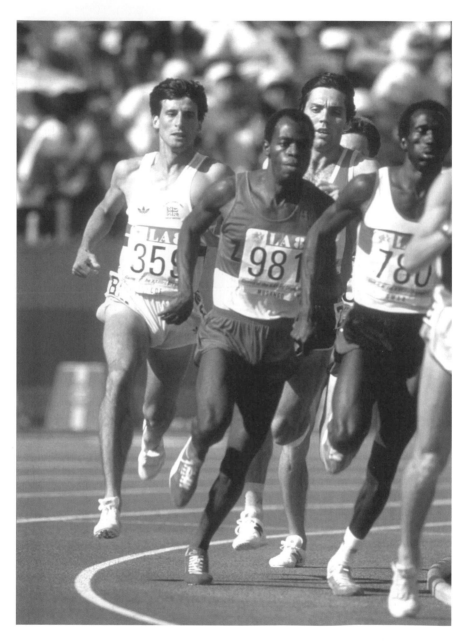

*Poised, connected and ready to pounce: Sebastian Coe (number 359)
during an 800 metres heat at the 1984 Los Angeles Olympic Games.*

If the runner I am trying to 'provoke' takes the bait and tries to show me and his colleagues who have heard my comment what he can really do, he is liable to forget everything he knows about form and just hammer that last 100. After he finishes, waving his arms around and trash-talking his mates, I will take this opportunity to point out to him that he put way more effort and unnecessary movement into that sprint than was really needed. This new information can be very useful in the runner's attempts to improve his form by helping him become aware of what he really does, as opposed to what he thinks he does. To reiterate Alexander's point, 'The most difficult things to change are those which "do not exist".'

If, on the other hand, the runner inhibits his reaction and maintains his good form while increasing his speed in an intelligent manner, this will serve him well when, for example, the need to accelerate presents itself in a race or perhaps to avoid an oncoming motorist.

So when your drill sergeant – I mean, coach – tries to provoke you, see how well you can keep your cool and your poise. With time, you will find that as your skill in these drills improves, so will your overall co-ordination.

● **To integrate good form – that is, good use – with good running mechanics.** Some drills are designed to highlight a certain phase in the stride cycle. For example, bum kicks are part of the forward swing phase in the cycle and high knees are part of the recovery or float period.

Coaches often use drills such as these to help runners develop a correct stride pattern. The problems arise when the emphasis is placed on the leg movement at the expense of the head-neck-back pattern. This is putting the cart before the horse, otherwise known as 'end-gaining'.

The Alexandrian runner will use drills as a stimulus to which he or she must learn to inhibit and direct. For example, when athletes do the high knees drill, they often lean backwards in the process. Try just lifting a knee parallel to the ground – you, too, may notice the urge to lean backwards. This is *not* required: the leg can move independently from the torso. So, rather than forcing the knee to come up to waist height, lift only as far as you can without disturbing the upward lengthening (verticality) of the torso (which you have initially engaged in your awareness prior to action). As your skill and flexibility increase, you will eventually be able to get it up, proper-like!

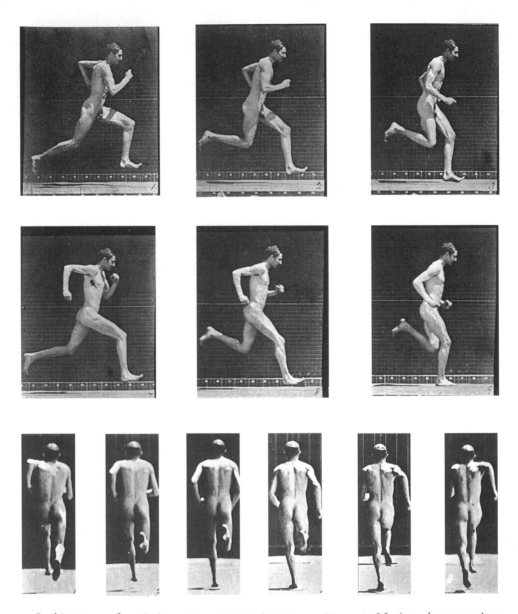

In this sequence from Eadweard Muybridge's The Human Figure in Motion, *the runner shows powerful use of the arms but a tendency to look down at the ground directly in front of him instead of into the middle distance.*

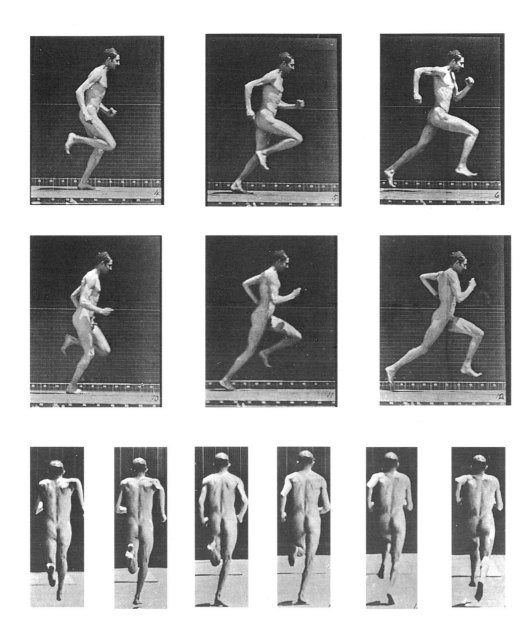

DRILLS FOR ALEXANDRIAN RUNNERS

● **High knees while avoiding neck tightening or spine shortening and maintaining your full length.** Ten seconds of running with the knees lifted so that your thigh is parallel to the ground. The challenge is to allow this to occur without 'losing the height', as my old coach, Bernard Godbout, used to exhort.

● **High knees at the bottom of a hill.** Repeat the above preventions and drill for five seconds at the bottom of a hill and then slowly run up the hill in short increments for ten seconds. I like to think of this as a moving lunge. It provides a strong stimulus for the athlete to maintain a sense of length in the torso. If this occurs, there is little or no sense of effort in the legs – just the opposite of what many runners experience going uphill. When done just before an acceleration, it can give a sense of effortless power. The reason is that the head and back are leading the movement and the legs are following, not the reverse.

● **Bum kicks.** Run slowly and allow your heels alternately to kick your bum. This drill should not be an excuse to arch the lower back and pull yourself down!

● **Accelerations.** Thirty seconds of accelerations alternated with 30-90 seconds of easy running can be done near the end of a long run. Don't leap into them, but take a little time to review your preventative directions first. When a runner accelerates using the legs, there is a tendency to stiffen the neck, lean backwards and shorten the torso – the exact opposite of what is required. When the runner inhibits this initial impulse but increases the rhythm of the arms, s/he will find that the legs follow suit – with less likelihood of disturbing the lengthening tendency of the spine.

● **Step-overs.** This is a drill I learned from Brent McFarlane, the Canadian national hurdles coach. I have found it a useful addition to my understanding of the concept of circularity in the running stride. It can help to develop a more efficient stride pattern and reduce wasted time and motion after the foot leaves the ground or toes off. It goes like this:

Having established the usual preventions, lift the right foot over and across the left ankle, and place the right foot back on the ground parallel to the left foot – not in front of it. Progress to stepping over the shin, and then over the knee.

This can be practised while standing still, walking, running slowly and then at full speed – and, of course, with the opposite leg. The challenge is to maintain a 'good attitude' at all times and not let the technical difficulty cause undue disturbance to the upthrust along the spine.

Like all the procedures outlined in this chapter, these drills can help runners improve their use if practised intelligently. Practised mechanically, they will only serve to reinforce existing patterns of misdirected effort and poor co-ordination.

SIX is fun for a running race.

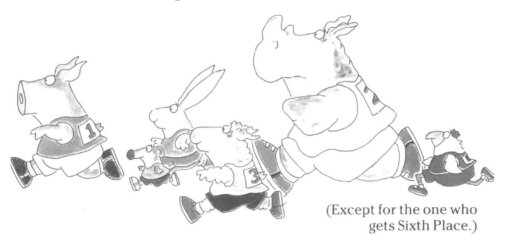

(Except for the one who gets Sixth Place.)

As we approach the chapter on competition, it's worth bearing in mind the message of this cartoon – and pondering George Sheehan's belief that 'when runners do their best, they are all equal'.

7. COMPETITION AND THE WINNING EDGE

Racing and other forms of competition are a natural continuation for people who have taken up running initially for some other reason. It gives us a chance to see how we measure up against the rest of the crowd. It can be an opportunity to put our training to a serious test. Or it might be the first step on the way to a place on the Olympic team.

Whatever the reason, competition can provide a strong source of motivation and inspire us to greater achievements, in terms of both performance and self-knowledge. It can also be a lot of fun.

In the Alexander world, there are at least two schools of thought on racing and competition. The first goes something like this: *avoid putting yourself in situations where you cannot inhibit your habitual responses in order not to compromise your newly-developed 'use'*. And there is much to be said for this approach. As someone once noted, 'You can't change and stay the same – alas!'

So for some people, taking a sabbatical from racing is necessary to break the negative patterns of tension and strain associated with the activity. In fact, running coaches generally agree that too much racing and competition can lead to impaired performance and burn-out.

Peter Coe told me that when his son Sebastian was at his peak, 14 or 15 races a year was the most he could take part in and stay competitive. From an Alexandrian perspective, we want the dog to wag the tail and not the other way around, and competition can be a very strong tail for the competitive runner. However, taking some time away from such a powerful stimulus can enable the athlete to pay attention in a way which is difficult – if not impossible – under competitive conditions.

As mentioned repeatedly, learning to 'inhibit' or refrain from the unwanted or unnecessary is the first step to making changes. The potential danger with this approach for the runner studying Alexander Technique is that s/he can

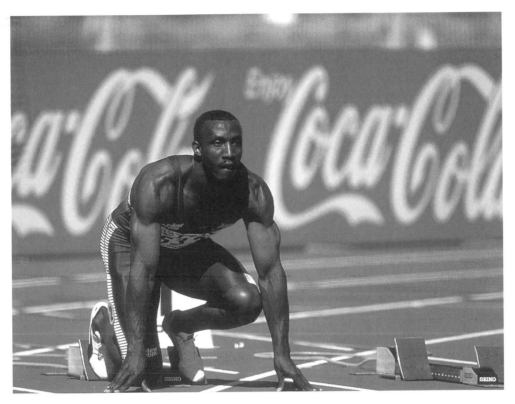

Linford Christie seeks the winning edge as he completes his mental rehearsal on the blocks at the 1995 World Championships.

develop a fear of going wrong. Working in the controlled environment that is the Alexander Technique lesson, where stimulation is reduced, reactions can be controlled more easily and 'use' improved – an ideal to which we can only aspire in real life. Trying to 'hold on' to these experiences, perhaps from fear of losing them, can lead to a state of paralysis.

This leads to the second school of thought, which can be described thus: *once you have learned how to 'think in activity', get out there and apply it.* Find the path, stray and find it again. If you stiffen your neck when you do 200 metres repeats, start to figure out how not to. As you get better at preventing this response, you will run better as well.

As a competitive person who has enjoyed pitting his strength, speed and skills against others since childhood, I have tried to find a balance between my competitive urges and my practice of the Alexander Technique. And I have come to the conclusion that the two are not incompatible. The challenge for me has been to learn to express my 'nature' in ways which don't unduly compromise my 'use'.

The chief danger with competition is that it can easily cause us blindly to seek the thrill of victory, while overlooking the inherent risks along the way. This is 'end-gaining'. However, as anyone who has tried this approach for very long finds out, in running at least, success takes time, patience and discipline. Trying for too much too soon is often a recipe for disaster.

Greed affects runners as much as it does stockbrokers. I vividly remember how this played out in my first marathon. Fuelled by the vision of breaking the three-hour barrier and the excitement of 15,000 people starting at the same time, I went out with the leaders and coasted through the first mile in just under five minutes. When I tell you that the last mile was completed in slightly over 13 minutes, including a very fast 'limp finish', you'll get the picture. And, no, I did not break three hours, or even three-and-a-half. It was a very painful lesson, which I only had to repeat two more times before it finally sunk in!

WINNING

'Everyone loves a winner,' so the saying goes. I like to win. So do most athletes. Unfortunately, winning has been championed by society, and specifically by marketing people in the shoe industry, as the *ultimate* measure of success in competition. For example, at the Atlanta Olympics, two slogans put out by major manufacturers went something like: 'Winning isn't everything, it's the only thing' and 'If you didn't come here for the gold you might as well have stayed home'. These make a complete mockery of the fantastic achievement just reaching the Olympics represents.

When you divide the world into winners (good) and losers (bad), it is clear what side most of us want to be on. However, there is only one actual winner in each race – so unless you are exceptionally talented or lucky then you're bound to be disappointed if winning is your only measure of success.

Instead, attempts have been made to redefine competition and winning. 'When runners do their best,' wrote George Sheehan, 'they are all equal. But the paradox is that those far back in the pack exceed the designated winners in the time they must endure the forces that would make them quit. So everyone is a hero. And none are more heroic than those deep in the flow of these struggles against time, distance and self'. Inspiring words, yet small consolation to those who long to be at the front of the pack with the 'real' winners.

Unless, that is, we alter our notions about the purpose of competition and what it means to be a winner. Winning does not always mean that we are the best, or even that we have done our best. You can win without being challenged, or without challenging yourself. You can also cheat in a race and win. However you can't cheat at what should arguably be the main goal of competition, namely 'to do your best against the rest'.

It's also important to note that unless you fix the outcome of the race, you can't control who wins. Even the best sometimes get beaten. Trying to control the uncontrollable is a great way to drive yourself and everyone around you nuts. So instead, looking at racing and competition through a different lens, we can shift our focus onto those things which are within our power to control, namely ourselves and our reactions. As Jerry Lynch noted in his excellent book *The Total Runner,* we need to focus on the process of the race, not just the outcome – what Alexander called the means rather than only the end. And Alexander Technique clearly shows us how we can develop this capacity in ourselves.

CHOICE

One of the key elements of Alexander Technique is the idea of choice: that little space between stimulus and response that we can learn to use to our advantage. Choice flavoured with clarity of intention, intelligence, courage and awareness can play a liberating role for the competitive runner.

There are lots of articles on how to avoid over-training, burn-out, injury and the like. Taking advantage of all this good advice is directly related to two of the key elements of Alexander Technique: namely our ability consciously to inhibit and direct. When we practise stopping and making intelligent decisions on a regular basis, it becomes a little easier to perform this act when the going gets tough. Reacting correctly in the heat of the race requires what I call 'presence', a quality which is directly related to how we are using ourselves in the moment.

PRESENCE

One of the interesting things about competition from an Alexandrian perspective is what you can learn about yourself and how you react in stressful situations. How well do you maintain, for example, your poise (that is, the integrity of the head-neck-back relationship)? Your clarity of intention? Your sense of perspective when you are overwhelmed with pre-race jitters? Your ability to maintain your grace under pressure?

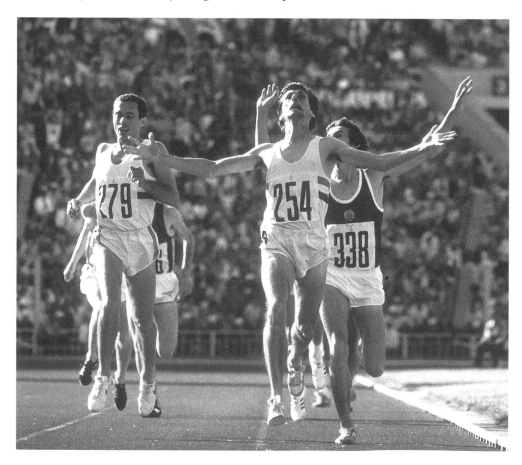

Exultation: after failing to win the 800 metres gold medal at the 1980 Moscow Olympics, Sebastian Coe (number 254) maintained his focus to beat old rival Steve Ovett in the 1,500 metres final.

Peter Coe, father of and coach to Sebastian, told me an interesting story about his son's failure to win the 800 metres gold medal at the Moscow Olympics. For those of you who weren't around then, Coe was the odds-on favourite for victory. He was the world record holder, in excellent shape, and was considered invincible over the distance. In Britain, the pressure on him to win was enormous, fulled by a press which has a habit of building up sports stars to such heights that failure to perform on the day is equated with high treason. Coe Senior recounted that his son seemed rather withdrawn on the morning of the race, noticeably quieter than usual. He did not comment on it at the time, because his style was to give an athlete enough room to run his own race. Except on this occasion he now knows it was a mistake. Coe's 'head was not in the race', and by the time he eventually woke up, another great British athlete, Steve Ovett, had too much of a lead for Seb to catch him. He was not close enough at the finish for his tremendous kick to make an impact and, in spite of an incredible effort, he finished second. For many people this would have been a great performance, but for Coe it was considered a disastrous failure.

A lot of the work I do as an Alexander Technique teacher is with musicians. One of the things I have noticed is that when musicians perform in public, they sometimes try and escape from their anxiety of the moment by disconnecting or hiding from the outside world. You can see it in their eyes: they aren't all there.

Rather than focusing on what lies ahead, all they want to do is get the hell out of there. The effect is that there is a difference in the quality of their performance. This is particularly true for singers, who have nowhere to hide. When this happens in an Olympic final, perhaps as a way of coping with the incredible pressure and expectation, the result is a lack of availability to respond appropriately to the situation at hand. In Coe's case, by the time he had reconnected, the damage had been done.

There is a second part to this story. Peter Coe recalls that he went against his custom when it came to the final of the 1,500 metres, and he gave Sebastian some rather direct advice about staying with the pace. He said, 'You stick so close to so-and-so that if he goes to the loo, you'll be in there handing him the paper' – or something to that effect! The upshot was that the overwhelming favourite to win the 1,500 metres, Steve Ovett, was beaten by Seb Coe – who did not lose his focus and was therefore in a position to use his kick to great effect.

A BALANCED APPROACH

During the Los Angeles Olympics, a number of athletes were asked hypothetically if they would be willing to take an undetectable drug which would guarantee them a gold medal but would greatly increase their risk of death within five years. An alarmingly high percentage said they would be prepared to do so.

In the book he wrote with his son, Peter Coe discussed the pros and cons of 'the running life'. While running is, for many, a rewarding experience full of joy and learning, for some 'it assumes the proportions of a religion or, worse still, becomes an addiction and an obsession. Its victims become unbalanced and hooked on mileage mania. From there, running can all too easily become a substitute for living and a retreat from the real world. Far from achieving the fitness and sense of well-being that it should bring, it is more likely to end in a frustrating crop of over-use injuries and a lowered level of health from constant over-stress'.

In contrast to these examples, I am writing from the perspective of someone who has learned to deal with competition in what I consider to be a slightly more balanced way than I once did. I used to think of a race purely in terms of my time, or whether I could finish ahead of a particular individual. I would get so nervous I could barely make it to the starting line. Given the level at which I competed, it all now seems rather silly; but at the time, it was close to being a matter of 'do or die'. Perhaps it is more a function of the ageing process, but I no longer allow that overpowering need to prove something to control my decision-making.

I now compete much less often than I used to, mostly because I don't want to race if I'm not prepared or, more importantly, if I'm not going to enjoy the experience. And that includes the discomfort which comes with pushing your limits.

WARMING-UP AND USE OF SELF

I recently had the interesting experience of running a race and the race finishing before I had a chance to catch up. I got lost on the way to the venue and arrived just ten minutes before the start, with nine other athletes to look after. By the time I had changed and handed the athletes their numbers on the starting line, the race was ready to begin. The gun went off and so did I — holding my number scrunched up in my right hand.

During the race, I noticed a number of things. First, I was really pumped-up: adrenalin was flowing big-time, mostly from the earlier worry that we would fail to make it in time to compete. This alone was enough to propel me through the first 800 metres in a blind rush: it was simply a matter of 'put it in gear and go'. Although I had run the course before, I kept thinking, 'Oh my God, we're at the hill already', or 'Yes, that was the fast bit where I should speed up', and so on. I kept hoping that something would slow down and let me catch up but, alas, it was me that slowed down and I never caught up.

This experience was a marked contrast from what usually occurs when I race. Normally I arrive an hour or so in advance, register and then jog slowly around the course. This gives me a chance to see how the route is set up, note any changes, and plan my race strategy. The last would include giving myself mental reminders, such as 'push the pace here', 'use my arms more before and after the hill to gain and maintain momentum', 'take this corner a bit wide so I don't lose speed', 'shorten my stride through the sandy bit', 'keep looking ahead', and so on. I would then take time to stretch and do mobility exercises, followed by some accelerations. Each phase of the preparation is designed to bring me (my *self*) to a state where I am ready to run fast.

The funny thing is that when I go through this kind of detailed rehearsal, the race doesn't seem fast. I have put myself in a position to anticipate, decide and execute rather than simply react. For example, I am not shocked by the hill suddenly appearing 'out of nowhere': I am ready for it and I know what to do. As a result, I am better able to maintain my form and consequently don't slow down as much. I feel as if I have more space and time to be aware of the wider context of the race – spectators, other runners, the weather – and still be able to attend to myself. This allows me to make the many small adjustments that can mean the difference between a good performance and a mediocre one. Most important of all, I have the experience that all of me is in the race and I am not merely trying to catch up with my legs.

ENDS VERSUS MEANS

In the 100 metres final at the 1999 World Championships, the great Canadian sprinter Bruny Surin made a tremendous start and was leading the field at the halfway mark. But at this point, Surin said afterwards, he panicked and tightened then tried to accelerate.

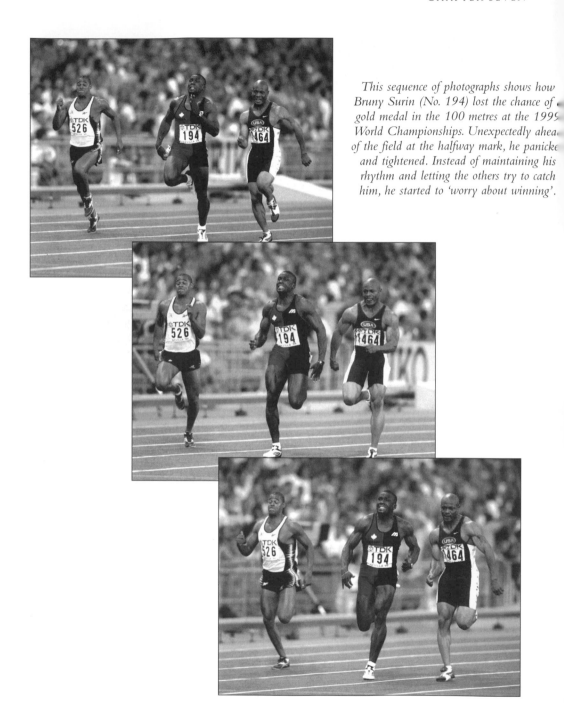

This sequence of photographs shows how Bruny Surin (No. 194) lost the chance of gold medal in the 100 metres at the 1999 World Championships. Unexpectedly ahead of the field at the halfway mark, he panicked and tightened. Instead of maintaining his rhythm and letting the others try to catch him, he started to 'worry about winning'.

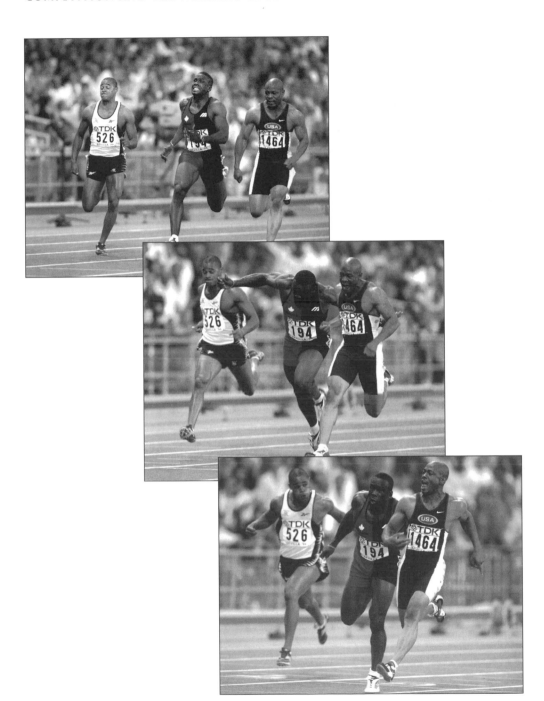

The cost of such a tiny distraction in world-class sprinting can be very high, given that the difference between the top competitors is mere tenths of a second. His coach, Michel Portmann, was watching the race from the sidelines and saw Surin's head pull back at this point. The world record holder, America's Maurice Greene, was then able to pass him and reach the line first. According to Portmann, there was no need for Surin to accelerate at that point; he simply needed to maintain his rhythm… and let the rest of the field try and catch *him*. Instead, he started to worry about winning. It was his momentary focus on this idea, rather than staying with 'the plan', that caused his downfall. Like Alexander, he needed to forget about winning, yet continue to do the things that would allow him to win – no small order under the circumstances.

Sprinters are taught to visualise their lane as a tunnel, in order to help shut out the potential distractions of rivals, officials and the crowd. The problem in this example is that when something managed to intrude into the imaginary tunnel, Surin's reaction was similar to the 'startle response' (a reflexive reaction to a sudden loud noise such as a door slam or gunshot which involves a strong contraction of the neck and other muscles and shortening of the stature). He tightened his neck, disrupting the poise of his head, which in turn affected his focus and rhythm. Attempting to correct his reaction by accelerating led to a general disturbance in his overall co-ordination.

Even if Surin had not panicked, Maurice Greene might have beaten him anyway. But speaking as a loyal Canadian, I don't think so!

RACING, FITNESS AND END-GAINING

To urge competitiveness and to urge caution in quick succession is not a contradiction. The longer you keep running well, the longer you will stay well. And if you are running for fitness, anything that curtails your running also curtails your fitness.

But lasting success has never been achieved without understanding the need for moderation. When applying increasing doses of stress – for that is what a large part of race training is – giving the correct opportunities for recovery requires careful thought. And if the top performers can practise restraint in their training build-up, then so can fitness runners, for certainly the same pressures are not on them.

Peter and Sebastian Coe

When runners first start competing, they sometimes go through a wonderful period where races bring a stream of personal-best performances. This is very reinforcing: instant reward for the effort expended. Alas, it soon passes, and a personal-best becomes more and more difficult to achieve.

When improvement starts to come more rarely, many runners become disillusioned and quit. They haven't learned, as George Leonard puts it, 'to love the plateau'.

As a coach, I try to encourage my athletes to 'stick with the programme'. In other words, to believe that following the training schedule will enable them to reach their goals. Yet some runners find it very difficult to hang in there day after day, allowing time for the adaptations to training to take place. They have what I call a 'High School mentality'.

In Canada every May or June, near the end of the academic year, many High Schools have a track and field meeting. Runners prepare for this event for two or three weeks and, on the big day, those with the most natural athletic talent win all the medals and get all the glory. This creates an illusion about what is really required for them to develop their potential. Arriving at university, the next step up where *everyone* has talent, requires a commitment to train 11 months of the year. The sacrifices needed to be competitive at this level come as a shock to their system.

British runners might like to think about the difference between being a star at schools level and making the step up to county or inter-club and league competition.

INJURIES

Injured runners are as common as flies in a horse barn. In *The New Competitive Runner's Handbook*, Bob Glover makes the following declaration: 'Like other athletes, competitive runners must learn to accept the inevitability of injury and illness. It is safe to say that every year of competitive running will find you injured or ill at least a few times'. The reality of this statement is echoed by another well-known runner/author, Jeff Galloway, who reckons that in his 25-year career he suffered more than one hundred lay-offs.

As a marathoner in the late 1970s, I suffered a wide variety of injuries and found myself constantly climbing out of the valley of rehabilitation. Looking back on that period now, I can't remember a time when I wasn't nursing a physical problem of some kind, in addition to the colds and flus that always seem to attack competitive athletes. Imagine my surprise when, after I began training as an Alexander Technique teacher in 1981, I no longer seemed to get hurt. In fact, from 1982 to 1999 (when I pulled a groin muscle trying to be a sprinter!), I did not suffer a single injury in spite of training and competing as an 800/1,500 metres runner. I'm not talking about the little niggles and aches that accompany any hard physical effort, but the kind of problem which involves time away from the track, physiotherapy or some other treatment and a period of rebuilding.

And it wasn't because I was babying myself. Anyone who has had the pleasure of training with Frank Horwill, as I have, will know that he doesn't pull any punches in his workouts. So what was making the difference?

There is a Zen saying: 'When the pupil is ready, the teacher arrives'. One day on the track, quite by chance (or so it seemed), I met Bernard Godbout, a coach in Montreal who told me I needed to learn how to run. I was both insulted and intrigued. What the hell was he on about? I'd finished five marathons and clocked up thousands of miles – I knew how to run. In fact, I had developed an ultra-efficient marathon shuffle, with a pronounced heel strike, tight arms and a tendency to sit on my legs. It didn't feel like that, of course: I thought I was running like Frank Shorter. But when I saw myself on video, I was shocked. Bernard was right: there was room for improvement. The seed had been planted and I knew that, in order to get faster, my form required a major overhaul.

Did I make a connection between running form and injuries at the time? Absolutely not. Initially, it was all about learning to run faster. It was only later that I realised this was an important step towards injury-free running. I think in hindsight that, like many, I had assumed running was a natural activity. It was simply a matter of buying a good pair of shoes and getting in shape: I had been a pretty decent ice hockey player so becoming a runner was simply a matter of putting in the miles. I never thought to consider that running might be 'natural' for an Ethiopian or a Kenyan because that was how they got to school or visited their neighbours. My basic modes of transport, in contrast, were bike, bus or car.

Why is this important? Consider the following. Biomechanical research indicates that in running, impact forces are three to five times greater than in walking. An average runner will take between 150-200 steps per minute. For someone who completes a marathon in 3 hr 20 mins at a rate of 160 strides per minute, this means he or she will make more than 32,000 impacts. Add the hundreds of training miles and the burning ambition to break the three-hour barrier and you have a recipe for disaster.

One of the benefits of taking Alexander Technique lessons is the awakening of what I call the 'kinaesthetic conscience'. This means that you start to notice how you do things and how much effort you put into them. For runners, this means discovering things like foot placement and how hard you land, breathing patterns, shoulder tension, sitting on the legs, and so on – in other words, you become much more aware of all the things that books and magazines tell you not to do but which you were too busy to heed.

During my training to become an Alexander Technique teacher, I became extremely motivated to prevent a recurrence of the many problems that had plagued my running. One of the few things I was capable of doing in the early stages was to pay attention, to observe what I was doing to myself when I ran. Not only did this make running more interesting, but it meant that I was beginning to pick up potential problems at an early stage. In addition, whereas before I was mainly concerned with such factors as how far, how fast and how often, my mental checklist now included how easy, how free and how smooth.

To say that runners can be irrational is a major understatement. Take, for example, the fact that there are marathon best-performance records from the age of six upwards. That one well-known athlete set a world record by running every day for 25 years. That a friend running the length of the Thames for charity, while suffering from achilles tendonitis severe enough to require his leg to be encased in plaster for more than a week when it was over, covered 60 miles in the last two days. The list goes on.

As for me, I often trained when I was injured, didn't take enough time for sufficient rest, ran in minus-35 degree weather, and so on – all to break three hours for the marathon. When viewed from a distance this looks crazy, but at the time it seemed perfectly normal – in fact, it was more the rule than the exception. I recently worked with a man in his early 40s, who ran a half-marathon in 72 minutes when aged in his 30s but was no longer able to run at all because of severe sciatica. He told me that of the 12 athletes with whom he trained in his 20s and 30s, none was still running: injuries had claimed them all. I have no doubt that I would be in the same position had I not stopped to reassess what I was doing and why, and decided on a different course of action.

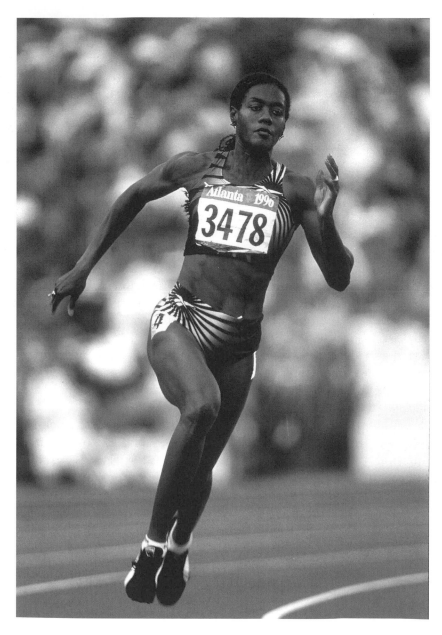

Merlene Ottey at the 1996 Olympic Games: efficient, graceful and powerful.

'USE' AND RUNNING MECHANICS

It is probably stating the obvious to say that learning to improve your stride – or what the exercise physiologist likes to call 'running mechanics' – is an advantage to the competitive athlete. Good mechanics help reduce the strain which competitive running places on the body; after all, the stresses that exist for the casual runner are multiplied many times for the racer. While the fun runner can choose to miss a race, the club or college athlete may find it much harder to duck a practice or bow out of a competition, especially when coaches, team-mates and supporters are counting on them.

The 'intelligent' runner can reduce the risk of injury by keeping total mileage down. However, the increased intensity of his or her 'quality' workouts will also increase the risk and potential cost of bad form or misdirected effort. As the level of competition gets tougher, so does the potential price one has to pay to stay in the game.

A second key reason for improving running mechanics is simply the matter of efficiency. The competitive athlete wants a maximum return on investment. S/he does not want to waste time or energy. Learning how to run so that energy/effort is translated as efficiently as possible into forward motion is indisputably important in competitive athletics. The reduction or elimination of unnecessary movement needs to be maximised, and the elements of an effective stride optimised. Some runners are born with the latter quality, but most can improve to some extent.

The learning process involved in improving our 'use' certainly helps with the development of a good stride. Runners with accurate sensory awareness can judge more clearly whether or not they are 'on track', and make adjustments accordingly.

A phrase often used in sport is 'in the zone'. It describes those fleeting moments when everything comes together, and you are able to perform at your peak with little or no gap between intention and actualisation. This is the holy grail for any athlete, and links back to the second of those Alexandrian schools of thought on competition. If you have learned how to 'think in activity', you have a far better chance of finding that elusive 'zone'.

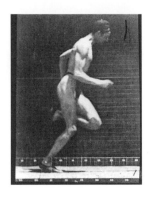

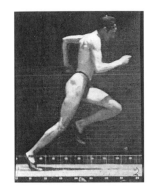

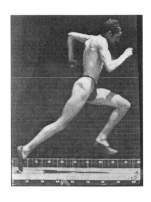

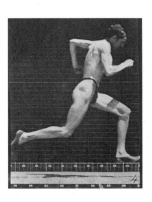

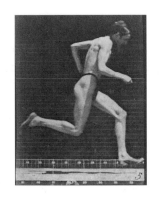

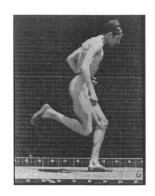

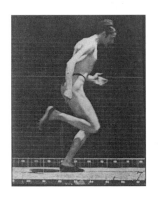

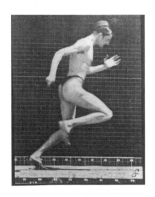

In this final sequence from Eadweard Muybridge's The Human Figure in Motion, *the runner is pushing his head forward with eyes looking directly down at the ground, causing him to tighten across the neck and shoulders.*

Afterword by John Woodward

'THE RUNNING SELF'

(John has for many years conducted 'natural running' workshops based on the principles of the Alexander Technique. The following testimony offers a glimpse of John's recent insights and experience with 'The Art of Running')

When Malcolm Balk asked me to write about my work with running and the Alexander Technique, his call came with an uncanny synchronicity. The previous day I had pledged to spend a whole year living and teaching strictly from within my own experience.

I had decided that I was up to here with information: overloaded. So in lessons and workshops I made it clear that there was no new information to take in, only that which individuals had brought with them. This meant not quoting from anybody else or referring to any other authority. It meant no diagrams, pictures or flip-charts, no passing people on to books or articles. It meant not writing anything down at all unless it was a poem to capture the particular flavour of a moment. So far, no-one has complained.

This piece began with a dilemma: should I write an objective piece about applying Alexander Technique to running skills, or should I see in the odd synchronicity a chance to crown the year-long exploration by creating a piece that goes into the experience of applying self-work to the activity of running? When I took this conundrum out on my favourite run, I was adamant about one thing: there is still too much information and I would take no delight in adding more to the excess.

This run from my Lakeland home takes in every kind of terrain and landscape. It begins along the sea-washed turf of the Duddon Estuary, which is perfect for barefoot running. It takes in a steep ascent of Kirkby Moor, through a small wood and along a green track to where the top of the moor opens to the Lakeland Hills and the estuary. There I descend through my village to return home. You are invited along on the run – it's uphill most of the way. When I reach the top there is a peak experience (forgive the pun) that runners sometimes call 'runners' high'. Here, the action freeze-frames in the turning step to begin the homeward descent.

Ancient cave-dwellers produced stunning wall pictures but evidently took little interest in their art thereafter. All the interest was in creating the picture. Runners would understand this better than most, because running is one of the few remaining avenues of modern culture with a natural, direct access to experience in its expression: the energy and rhythm of words, strides and sentences are inextricably intertwined.

Running. The first step: begin. The final step: begin again. Each stride is subtly different from the last one and the next one. I'm digging in now, to pull up the slope leading to the edge of Kirkby Moor. With the wind up like this, white-horse waves of the Irish Sea should be visible from the north tip of Walney Island. Running is so much about timing, cycles and rhythms – as in nature, where the tides ebb and flow, the moon waxes and wanes, the Earth spins through the changing seasons.

I need more oxygen to fuel my muscles to get me up this rise. There is an oxygen debt. The breath expands and its rhythm quickens to the demand, the blood delivering oxygen to every cell, the breath touching every corner in the fabric of my running body. A pulse has its peaks and troughs, lifts and falls. The pulse of life never varies, but the rhythms constantly shift and change: sometimes slow, sometimes quick, sometimes smooth, sometimes jerky. These running legs work to their cycle: this one is weight-bearing, while the other releases and lifts, before dropping through a pendulum arc to place my foot to rest briefly on the moorland turf, balancing the body above, before driving me on into this westerly wind. The lift and fall of the cycle of my running legs never varies, but the rhythm does – sometimes leading with the left leg, sometimes with the right. Sometimes the cadence is fast, sometimes it is slow, sometimes the stride length is long, sometimes short. The rhythm needs shifting to match the varying terrain.

Now I need a second wind to get up this steady incline with a westerly wind blowing straight into my face. There's a lot of pain to be penetrated and overcome in running. Perhaps that's the hell of it. But then there is always the third wind of the runner's high: the heaven of it. I wonder if the runner's high is the way that the brain signals to the body its approval of higher levels of integration, a kind of endorphin endorsement of the rhythms and cycles of mind and body coming together in rich, resonating harmony. No wonder we chase after it.

There are 'Turk's heads' immediately up ahead. This is the local name for capricious tussocks of long grass strewn among the stretch of purple moorland. Until your foot has landed into the tussock, there's no knowing how a Turk's head will deal with you. This one tips me over to the left and requires an instant throwing out of the right arm to maintain balance. I only just got away with it this time; I was thinking too much about runner's high and not paying enough attention to the demands of the moment – the perennial error.

I am entering Peppers Wood now, and there is a special challenge left by the cycle of the seasons. The scattered autumn leaves mask slatey stones beneath. And there's too much light and shade for my eyes to read the path ahead and feed the information to my body. I've been in this situation before and I've run with complete self-abandon, going at full tilt, trusting my feet to see, to sort out the crackling leaves from the sharp stones. Letting go. Trusting. But this is not the right moment. So I rein back to a walking step and give my eyes a chance to marvel at the endless variety of leaves.

I am looking down now at my running body as I pick up the pace and leave the gate out of Peppers Wood behind me. I can look at my moving body as an object, and the body is indeed a mechanism with its rods and levers, pulleys, valves, pipework and pumps. This rhythmically pulsing mechanism of a body cleaves itself through the air. The tendency is to want to scrunch down into this head-on wind, to do battle with it, to think about it impeding my forward progress. But I have found a rhythm now. My running body ploughs through the air like the prow of a ship. This rhythm is good, but watch out! Here the ground is boggy, with a thin covering of slimy vegetation coating vertically-stacked, razor-sharp strata of the Skiddaw slate that forms the massive bulk of Kirkby Moor. A slip on this, a loss of balance, one foot jamming down hard to recover, can lead to the hell of being laid-up with an injury. I decide not to pull back but to open up, to allow for more degrees of freedom, a greater refinement of balance and adjustment to match the uncertain nature of the terrain. Stride length shortens, cadence increases to maintain maximum security of foot-plant while running speed increases slightly. Is it the adrenalin or an endorphin rush? It's like flying to go so completely with my nature in this way.

Deep inside the experience of moving over the beautiful Lakeland landscape, I begin to wonder about the subtle but distinct difference between my running body and my running self. I am looking down at the mechanical thrust-bars, the levers of the leg bones, and the pull-machines of the muscles that move them over this varied terrain. Seeing my body as an external object is distinct from the experience of my running self. This sense of being alive right now is certainly as real as these pumping arms and driving legs. Curious how often people try to explain the experience of the runner's high in terms of feeling intensely alive and yet no-one can point a finger at the experience. In its very subjectivity it takes the form of self-knowing. The objective world deals with the world out there, while the subjective world deals with the self, the world in here, the experience of which must be the basic source of all my learning.

There is a fork in the track. Which way to go? Up ahead, the windmills atop Kirkby Moor turn incessant cartwheels in the strong westerly. They seem to beckon me to the summit. Where have I been? Where am I going? Where am I now? The way ahead for my running self peels out of the present living moment and into a perpetual fork in the road ahead. There is the road well-worn and the way less-trodden. It is an ongoing game while I am running along: to put up signposts at the fork in the road ahead of my running self and, although the paths fork in the same way, I like to write different destinations on the signposts.

To run naturally is to run with life. To run mechanically is to run with the drudgery of deadness, the hell of being locked outside the living experience which is the very fabric of self-knowledge. And so I label the path well-trod: 'To Mechanical Running via the way of Habit'. The other track, the less-worn route, I label: 'To Natural Running via the way of Unhabit'. Human beings do have a choice in the perpetual fork in the road ahead. Much hangs on that choice.

Not too far back in the bow-wave of my past is the time I spent with Paul Collins, who died five years ago. Paul seems very alive in this moment. I can feel his fingers on my neck. I had lessons with Paul that you could count on my two hands. Although I did not train to be an Alexander teacher with Paul, I regarded him as my teacher. Here on top of Kirkby Moor, the inspiration of this master runner is powerfully present.

I was there when Paul took what would turn out to be his final running steps before he died. The occasion was at the end of the third, week-long summer course on running and the Alexander Technique. He demonstrated then the highest levels of self-mastery. From the outside it was an awkward, shambling last run. Paul never looked that good in his running style: he had made too many adjustments and compensations in order to overcome the injuries that ended his early competitive running career. But what was happening on the inside of that last running mile, to overcome the pain and fatigue of the cancer that eventually killed him, was a triumph of self-direction and an ongoing inspiration to me.

Paul ran his last mile as if it were the first, with new conditions to overcome and new beginnings to negotiate. More and more towards the end of his life, he became intrigued by the significance of taking one fully aware step. For him, the effort of making that single aware step would easily weigh down the scales against the effort of taking a billion habit-locked, mechanical steps. As the future of the self peels into the perpetual fork, the way less-trod leads to the attainment of a beginner's mind. I learned from Paul's inspiration that having made the effort to get into the Way of Unhabit, you begin again. It is a cycle – and running, like life itself, is all about rhythm, cycles and new beginnings.

Dr Rob Greaves got a sense of breaking into the inside of running when he wrote in evaluation of a course: 'I am astounded. How can I have been doing something for almost 50 years and yet know so little about myself?' There is an openness and humility in Rob's words. He is a hard-headed, no-nonsense medical man who is trained to be objective. Rob's testimony grows out of that extraordinary effort to run onto the path less-trod, and as a result Rob got inside his self. You can hear in his statement shock and consternation, tinged with not a little despair. Rob is a diligent, intelligent and committed runner. He had been working hard on his running, but from the outside. The effort of making it onto the inside is the crucial first step towards 'natural running'.

On the course, I often begin by putting to runners the honest question: 'Why run? Why do you do it?'. The answers that come back are about as varied as the individuals: to get more physically fit; to run away (particularly from the pressures and stresses of work); to run towards something (such as the goal of a sub-three hour marathon); to get from A to B; to beat an existing record or personal-best time; to run into creative or imaginary landscapes.

These are a representative sample of answers, all valid reasons to run, all very reasonable goals to be achieved. The difficulty is that it is quite possible to be caught in a mechanical loop and yet still have the pervasive illusion of getting somewhere. After all, distances are covered, probably gaining cardio-vascular fitness as the miles are clocked up; stresses of work or relationships are shaken down; personal-best times and distances may be achieved and escapes into creative landscapes can be realised. But still it can be like a carousel, a merry-go-round with an illusion of real movement, when all that is actually happening is a coursing around on the spot. Attaining the listed goals may even reinforce a locked-up and locked-outside quality. This will be equally, if not more, true for the naturally talented athlete than for us less-gifted and struggling. The inevitable end result of getting fit via mechanical running is a locking-up within our physical structure, a fixity within the loop of existing habits and a holding-on to the limits of the known and the safe. Actually there is no truth that way, and no true sport either. There is a characteristically grim Lancashire expression that goes, 'If you rattle up and down the same niche for long enough it will dig a trench six feet deep and they can lower your coffin into it'. To clamber out of the trench requires a particular effort.

I often heard Paul say that 'the ideal Alexander Technique is what would happen in nature if there were no interference'. Here the emphasis is on a negative, on a process of subtraction, taking away the hindrances that interfere with a freer, more natural movement. This effort is not all of everything, but it is the start of everything concerning self-work. The size of the problem is reflected in Rob's plaintive words. He realised how easily the carousel of habit can go merrily round, often achieving the goals that runners list as the objectives of their running. The big difficulty is to realise, as Rob did, that it is not possible to get to know yourself better that way. Running does not have to be a form of self-study, though it turns out to be an excellent one.

Most participants on the 'natural running' course have an experience of the deeply serious nature of play, while at the same time appreciating the lightness, levity and wonderful paradox of it all. One described the course as being 'like running along a precipitous cliff at full tilt'. I would go along with her sense of risk and trust inherent in true play, only I would go even further and liken it to running flat out along an arête ridge – a balancing act in which if I lose it and fall over one way, I fall into the collapse of existential nothingness and despair. Whereas if I lose it the other way, I fall into the strain, effort and mind-numbing drudgery of work. Play is a tightrope act, a risky business – dangerous fun!

There is a sense of kinship generated on the week-long running courses which astonishes and delights me. After all, we are enthusiasts, amateurs who love what we do. Running can and should be a highly competitive sport, but that competitive spirit is further down the line. First there is the shared aim of getting more of the whole into the running that we do. We fundamentally share the very human endeavour of self-discovery. Running is a great source of fellow feeling, and the shared aim is to make the most of who and what we are. It is a great leveller, too. A particular delight is to bring together individuals from widely different backgrounds. Once Lennie, the hospital porter from Bermondsey, was roomed together with Laurie, the Harley Street psychiatrist. They got on famously, sharing a common commitment to self-work and self-discovery.

The exertion of energy to lift me up here to the top of Kirkby Moor physically stretches and extends my muscles. There is a flow of energy: an interchange between runner and nature and back again from nature to runner. The rhythmic thumping of my heart muscle is opened-out, expanded. Within the self, too, there has been an expansion of the heart: a passion to affirm my being in the world, to live this life to the full. After all, I can live no-one else's life! What I cannot find here in the pulsing energy of this living body I will find nowhere else. Consciousness is energy, and the search is all. I can only fully discover who I am by getting out into the world and discovering what I can do. But only by establishing the right order of priority can I bring the being and doing, the subject and object of my running, together in a constructive way: when first things come first and second things come second, there is order and integrity. When second things come first there is disarray and fragmentation.

A natural runner makes the transition from animal grace to human grace by placing first things first and second things second, and becomes a conscious automaton capable of seeing through habit. The mechanical runner puts the second things first and becomes an unconscious automaton. The step between a conscious automaton and a habit-locked unconscious automaton is both a very small step and a very great leap. It is a paradox.

As soon as self-work is brought to running, there is an immediate head-on confrontation with self-limiting patterns. This is tough work. For it to begin, the leash behind a habit-locked runner has to be pulled hard. This brings a mechanical runner to a juddering halt. Because second things are being put first, there is a twitchy drive to get on with the training runs, the exercise schedules, the injury analysis and the more competitive edge to performance. But hang on! These are all second things. First comes the pause, in order to examine whatever is preventing the whole of the self from entering the activity of running.

The preoccupation with achieving second things first has to be confronted for real self-work to begin. But when an individual runner makes the effort to put first things first, they take with them into action the all-important quality of stillness. Their running action has a quiet, centred grace and they run with complete self-acceptance, at ease with the uniqueness of their particular individual constitution. They are truly ready: prepared to train with an insight that will tailor exercise schedules to fit their needs, ready to fine-tune up to maximum performance for competition. There is a particular joy in seeing runners move with a freedom and rhythmic lilt as if they are animated from within by a hidden source of energy: consciousness. The crowning delight is to see how they all run differently, and the self-expression of running becomes an unfurling celebration of uniqueness, individuality and life.

There is a new lightness in the stride that leads me into the next step, downhill from Kirkby Moor. And the future, as it peels into the perpetual fork ahead, has a strong direction to continue writing this piece as an ongoing process of self-exploration. This is a challenge, with many attendant risks and vulnerabilities. But then, in the work of the self, the search is what really matters. Also, I take with me the inspiration of a true teacher. I now have a fuller appreciation of Paul Collins' preoccupation with the first fully-awake step. Paul brought insight and life to his running and teaching, because he made the effort to teach from his personal search and not from his knowledge. This means not disseminating information, but inspiring the process of self-discovery.

A text of written words easily becomes a dead body, detached from the energy of the search and the consciousness which is central to self-work. When I look now at these words, I see them as a shed skin. While I hope that the energy behind the words will help others in their search through the formless art of running, that hope must not blind me to the effort of letting go, beginning again and moving on into the next step.

OTHER SOURCES

Rodney Cullum & Lesley Mowbray: 'The English YMCA Guide to Exercise to Music' (Pelham, 1988)
Roger Golten: 'The Owner's Guide to the Body' (Thorsons, 1999)

A wealth of information about **Eadweard Muybridge** is available on the internet, with many sites offering animated sequences: the two best are www.linder.com/muybridge and www.kingston.ac.uk/muytext0.htm

USEFUL ADDRESS

The Society of Teachers of the Alexander Technique 20 London House, 266 Fulham Road, London SW10 9EL (020 7351 0828) www.stat.org.uk

PICTURE CREDITS

First published in Great Britain by
ASHGROVE PUBLISHING
an imprint of
HOLLYDATA PUBLISHERS LTD
55 Richmond Avenue
London N1 0LX

First edition

ISBN 1-85398-132-X

Book Design by Brad Thompson
Printed and bound in Malta by Interprint